Attention Deficit Disorder

Volume 3

Other related Pergamon titles of interest

BLOOMINGDALE & SWANSON

Attention Deficit Disorder: Volume IV Current Concepts and Trends in Attentional and Behavioural Disorders in Childhood

BLOOMINGDALE & SERGEANT

Attention Deficit Disorder: Volume V

Attention Deficit Disorder

Volume 3

NEW RESEARCH IN ATTENTION, TREATMENT, AND PSYCHOPHARMACOLOGY

Edited by

LEWIS M. BLOOMINGDALE

New York Medical College, Valhalla, New York, USA

Proceedings of the Third High Point Hospital Symposium on ADD, held 30 October–1 November 1983 at Sausalito, California and sponsored by The Gralnick Foundation

PERGAMON PRESS
OXFORD · NEW YORK · BEIJING · FRANKFURT
SÃO PAULO · SYDNEY · TOKYO · TORONTO

U.K.	Pergamon Press plc, Headington Hill Hall, Oxford OX3 0BW, England
U.S.A.	Pergamon Press Inc., Maxwell House, Fairview Park, Elmsford, New York 10523, U.S.A.
PEOPLE'S REPUBLIC OF CHINA	Pergamon Press, Room 4037, Qianmen Hotel, Beijing, People's Republic of China
FEDERAL REPUBLIC OF GERMANY	Pergamon Press GmbH, Hammerweg 6, D-6242 Kronberg, Federal Republic of Germany
BRAZIL	Pergamon Editora Ltda, Rua Eça de Queiros, 346, CEP 04011, Paraiso, São Paulo, Brazil
AUSTRALIA	Pergamon Press Australia Pty Ltd., P.O. Box 544, Potts Point, N.S.W. 2011, Australia
JAPAN	Pergamon Press, 5th Floor, Matsuoka Central Building, 1-7-1 Nishishinjuku, Shinjuku-ku, Tokyo 160, Japan
CANADA	Pergamon Press Canada Ltd., Suite No. 271, 253 College Street, Toronto, Ontario, Canada M5T 1R5

First edition 1988

Library of Congress Cataloging in Publication Data

High Point Hospital Symposium on ADD (3rd: 1983: Sausalito, Calif.)
Attention deficit disorder, volume 3: new research in treatment, psychopharmacology, and attention: the proceedings of the Third High Point Hospital Symposium on Attention Deficit Disorder, October 30–November 1, 1983, Sausalito, California/edited by Lewis M. Bloomingdale; introduction by Dennis P. Cantwell. 87-2446

British Library Cataloguing in Publication Data

Attention deficit disorder.
Vol. 3
1. Children, Brain. Minimal brain dysfunction
I. Bloomingdale. Lewis M. *1919–*
618.92'8589

ISBN 0-08-036466-7

Printed in Great Britain by A. Wheaton & Co. Ltd, Exeter

Preface

AT THE end of the first High Point Hospital Symposium on ADD, Keith Conners, Marcel Kinsbourne and I talked about the meeting on the way to the airport. Through the good offices of The Gralnick Foundation, I had been able to bring together a group of international experts doing research in ADD together for direct communication and all the participants wanted to continue these annually.

The true value of these symposia is to present to psychiatrists, neurologists, psychologists, pediatricians, and educators the results of years of scientific labor, papers at the cutting edge of research into the theory and practice of a fascinating entity, a simulacrum, perhaps, from one point of view, but an affliction that all of us know causes horrendous damage to the ADD child and his frustrated parents.

Even before the studies on adult Attention Deficit Disorder (ADD-R) were published, we all knew that this disorder could have malevolent sequelae in the adult who had suffered from the disorder in childhood. The high incidence of delinquency in prospective studies of ADD, the similarity of autonomic responses in the ADD child and psychopathic adults have yet to be thoroughly investigated but are addressed in this volume. The studies of the criminal population in prisons (especially sociopaths) by a questionnaire similar to that which Huessy developed for investigating the incidence of childhood ADD in alcoholics (Chapter 2, this volume) or by other screening tests, may indicate that a high percentage of prisoners with psychopathic personalities had ADD in childhood.

We remind the reader that the victims of psychopathic criminals and the costs to society of the legal processes and correctional institutionalization of such individuals is enormous in the US, and the rest of the world today. If a high percentage of children with Conduct Disorder become psychopaths as adults, the urgency of research in this field is of the utmost importance to society at large.

The shame of the ADD child with an IQ that is normal or above, particularly if there is concurrent Learning Disorder, is excruciating. The shame of the child's parents and the total consequent effect on the family constellation is painful at best and not infrequently chaotic. Probably the best treatment available for ADD children (and the expense renders this impractical for wide-scale application) is the combined intensive behavior therapy and psychostimulant medication described by Pelham in Chapter 3. Even this is still ineffectual in terms of social outcome.

The papers in this volume are impressive and represent years of research by a highly intelligent group of investigators who have presented their findings with appropriate caution. As exemplified in this and other volumes of this series, substantial advances have been made in theory and practice. However, we are in the position of a hiker climbing a mountain in the rarified, clear air of the Rockies. The peak always seems to be as far away as when we started; it is only when we look back that we can see how far we have come. In the areas of child neurology, child psychology, education, and all other professional disciplines involved in ADD or ADD-R, we have yet to find effective preventive treatment in the puerperium, parturition, infancy, or childhood of these children to alter the incidence of Conduct Disorder (and possibly delinquency and psychopathy). The Satterfields (Cf. Chapter 17) offer some hope. (For technical reasons and because 10-year follow-up results have been published,* Chapter 17 is summarized in this volume. *Editor*.)

If these High Point Hospital Symposia and this series of volumes contribute to the alleviation of the miseries of ADD children and their parents, and if theory leading to rational practice improves the diagnosis and prognosis of these "difficult children," the effort has been worthwhile.

LEWIS M. BLOOMINGDALE, M.D.

*Satterfield JH, Satterfield BT and Schell AM Therapeutic interventions to prevent delinquency in hyperactive boys. *J. Amer. Acad. Chil. & Adolesc. Psychiat.*, 1987, **26**: 56–64.

Acknowledgments

I WOULD like to express my appreciation for the initial funding by The Gralnick Foundation, High Point Hospital, Port Chester, New York, that enabled me to start and continue this series of High Point Hospital Symposia on Attention Deficit Disorder and to prepare these volumes for publication. I am grateful to the participants for their cooperation in the provision of manuscripts, re-editing of those, and their participation in the discussion of the papers presented.

Mrs Marie O'Leary has been invaluable in the arrangements for these symposia and, in particular, for her many hours of work, often late at night, to meet deadlines, in the preparation of the manuscripts. I am indebted to her for the contribution to ADD research she has made by her efforts.

LEWIS M. BLOOMINGDALE, M.D.

Apologia

I WOULD like to thank all of the contributors to this volume for submitting promptly articles based upon the talks they gave at the Third High Point Hospital Symposium, held in Sausalito, California, in 1983.

Unfortunately, Spectrum Publications, that had agreed to publish this series of volumes, ran into difficulties beyond anyone's control and the copy for the volume languished in a corrected, computerized format. Eventually, our publishers went out of business and the series will henceforward be published by Pergamon Press.

It was necessary to condense the volume, both because of publishing requirements and in view of the fact that several chapters had been published in an updated version, making those authors' chapters obsolete.

Accordingly, we have replaced these articles (marked by a dagger) with a one-page précis with references to the updated material published for the reader's use.

We regret that publication problems prevented a timely release of this volume and I thank those contributors who consented to having their papers omitted from this volume.

LEWIS M. BLOOMINGDALE, M.D.

Contents

Contributors

GEORGE M. ANDERSON, Ph.D.—Assistant Professor of Laboratory Medicine, Yale University School of Medicine, New Haven, Connecticut.

MARY E. BENDER, M.A.—Clinical Psychologist, Department of Psychiatry, University of California, Irvine, California.

AGNETA D. BORGSTEDT, M.D.—Clinical Professor of Pediatrics (Neurology), University of Rochester School of Medicine and Dentistry, Rochester, New York.

MAURICE BOUDREAULT, M.D., C.S.P.G., L.M.C.C.—Professor, Department of Psychiatry, Laval University, Quebec, Canada.

MARY SUE BUDROW, M.A.—School Psychologist, Lewiston City Schools, Lewiston, Idaho.

D. B. BYLUND, Ph.D.—Associate Professor of Pharmacology, Pharmacology Department, University of Missouri, Columbia, Missouri.

DENNIS P. CANTWELL, M.D.—Joseph-Campbell Professor of Child Psychiatry, and Director of Residency Training in Child Psychiatry, University of California at Los Angeles, Neuropsychiatric Institute, Los Angeles, California.

PHILIPPE CÁPERAÁ, Ph.D.—Professor, Department of Mathematics, Faculty of Sciences, Laval University, Quebec, Canada.

DONALD J. COHEN, M.D.—Professor of Pediatrics, Psychiatry and Psychology, Yale University School of Medicine; Director, Yale Child Study Center, New Haven, Connecticut.

ROBERT CÔTÉ, Ph.D.—Professor, Department of Mathematics, Faculty of Sciences, Laval University, Quebec, Canada.

J. W. EARL, Ph.D.—Biochemist, Department of Pathology, Royal Alexandra Hospital for Children, Sydney, Australia.

RANDALL W. EVANS, Ph.D.—Research Fellow, Biological Sciences Research Center, University of North Carolina School of Medicine, Chapel Hill, North Carolina.

H. BRUCE FERGUSON, Ph.D.—Professor, Department of Psychology, Carleton University; Adjunct Professor of Psychiatry, Faculty of Health Sciences, University of Ottawa, Ottawa, Ontario, Canada.

JUDITH VAN WYCK FLEET—Clinical Research Scientist, Psychiatry Section, Medical Division, Burroughs Wellcome Co., Research Triangle Park, North Carolina.

ROBERT D. GLASER, M.A.—Research Assistant, Department of Psychology, University of Missouri, Columbia, Missouri

C. THOMAS GUALTIERI, M.D.—Associate Professor of Psychiatry, Research Scientist, Biological Sciences Research Center, University of North Carolina School of Medicine, Chapel Hill, North Carolina.

LILY HECHTMAN, M.D. (F.R.C.P.)—Associate Professor, Department of Psychiatry and Assistant Professor, Department of Pediatrics, McGill University, Montreal, Quebec, Canada.

ROBERT E. HICKS, Ph.D.—Research Associate Professor of Psychiatry, Research Scientist, Biological Sciences Research Center, University of North Carolina School of Medicine, Chapel Hill, North Carolina.

CHRISTIANE M. HOPPE, Ph.D.—California State University, Long Beach, California.

ELLEN HORWITZ, Ph.D.—Clinical Assistant Professor, Department of Psychiatry, University of Missouri, Columbia, Missouri.

DAVID C. HOWELL, Ph.D.—Professor of Psychology, University of Vermont College of Medicine, Burlington, Vermont.

HANS R. HUESSY, M.D.—Professor of Psychiatry, University of Vermont, College of Medicine, Burlington, Vermont.

ROBERT D. HUNT, M.D.—Assistant Professor of Psychiatry, Yale University School of Medicine, Yale Child Study Center; Director of Child and Adolescent Services, West Haven Mental Health Clinic and Connecticut Mental Health Center, New Haven, Connecticut.

JAVAID JAVAID, Ph.D.–Assistant Director, Biological Research Laboratory, Illinois State Psychiatric Institute, Chicago, Illinois.

L. JOHNSTON, B.A.—Psychologist, Sydney Catholic Church Schools, Sydney, Australia.

MARCEL KINSBOURNE, M.D.—Chairman, Department of Behavioral Neurology, Shriver Center, Waltham, Massachusetts; Lecturer in Neurology, Harvard Medical School and Massachusetts General Hospital, Boston Massachusetts; Adjunct Professor, Department of Psychology, Brandeis University, Waltham, Massachusetts.

RAFAEL KLORMAN, Ph.D.—Professor of Psychology and Psychiatry, Director of Clinical Training, University of Rochester, Rochester, New York.

DAVID A. MARKS, Ph.D.—Department of Psychology, Washington State University, Pullman, Washington.

MICHEL MAZIADE, M.D., C.S.P.Q., F.R.C.P., L.M.C.C.—Child Psychiatrist, Professor, Department of Psychiatry, Laval University, Quebec, Canada.

JAMES MILLER, M.A.—School Psychologist, Moscow City Schools, Moscow, Idaho.

RUUD B. MINDERAA, M.D.—Child Psychiatrist, Sophia Kinderziekenhuis, Rotterdam, The Netherlands.

DAVID E. NILSSON, Ph.D.—Adjunctive Psychologist, Primary Children's Hospital, Salt Lake City, Utah.

CAROL PALUCHOWSKI, M.A.—Department of Child and Family Studies, Washington State University, Pullman, Washington.

KENNERLY PATRICK, Ph.D.—Research Associate, Biological Sciences Research Center, University of North Carolina School of Medicine, Chapel Hill, North Carolina.

WILLIAM E. PELHAM, Ph.D.—Associate Professor, Department of Psychology, Florida State University, Tallahassee, Florida.

HERBERT C. QUAY, Ph.D.—Professor of Psychology and Pediatrics, University of Miami, Coral Gables, Florida.

MARILYN RONNEI, M.A.—Department of Psychology, Washington State University, Pullman, Washington.

LEONARD F. SALZMAN, Ph.D.—Professor of Psychiatry (Psychology), Associate Chairman, Department of Psychiatry, University of Rochester School of Medicine and Dentistry, Rochester, New York.

BREENA SATTERFIELD, M.S.—Clinical Faculty, UCLA School of Medicine, Los Angeles, California.

JAMES H. SATTERFIELD, M.D.—Research Director, National Center for Hyperactive Children, Encino, California.

ANNE M. SCHELL, Ph.D.—Department of Psychology, Occidental College, Los Angeles, California.

ROBERT W. SCHNEDLER, Ph.D.—Clinical Psychologist, Sacred Heart Medical Center, Spokane, Washington.

G. L. SERFONTEIN, M.B., ChB., F.C.P. (S.A.)—Consultant Paediatrician, Royal Alexandra Hospital for Children, Sydney, Australia.

JOSEPH SERGEANT, Ph.D.—Senior Lecturer in Experimental and Clinical Psychology, Laboratory for Experimental Clinical Psychology, State University, Gröningen, The Netherlands.

WALID O. SHEKIM, M.D.—Associate Professor of Psychiatry, University of Missouri, Columbia, Missouri.

JOVAN G. SIMEON, M.D.—Professor, Department of Psychiatry, Faculty of Medicine, University of Ottawa, Ottawa, Ontario.

JAMES M. SWANSON, Ph.D.—Professor of Pediatrics and Psychiatry, University of California, Irvine, California College of Medicine, Orange, California.

JACQUES THIVIERGE, M.D., C.S.P.Q., F.R.C.P.—Professor of Child Psychiatry, Department of Psychiatry, Laval University, Quebec, Canada.

RONALD L. TRITES, Ph.D.—Professor of Psychiatry and Psychology, University of Ottawa, Ottawa, Ontario.

GABRIELLE WEISS, M.D. (F.R.C.P.)—Professor of Psychiatry, Department of Psychiatry and Associate Professor of Pediatrics, Department of Pediatrics, McGill University, Montreal, Quebec, Canada.

Introduction

IT IS a pleasure to introduce this volume, the third in a series of the proceedings of a two-day symposium in which active investigators in the field of ADD were brought together under the leadership of Lewis M. Bloomingdale, M.D., to discuss their findings and to stimulate new research.

Over a decade ago, I published a six-stage model that I felt could be useful for the study of all psychiatric disorders of childhood, consisting of the following: First, a clear description of the clinical picture the child presents, including the essential and the significant associated features of the disorder. The second stage consists of physical and neurologic factors. The third stage involves family studies of two types: family illness studies and family interaction. Family illness studies are studies of the prevalence and type of psychopathology in close relatives of the index probands, while family interaction studies are studies of the interaction between family members and the proband.

The fourth phase involves laboratory studies, which could be electrophysiologic, neuroendocrine, biochemical; all of which would be etiologic in nature, or, in considering ADD, measures of attentional mechanisms and activity levels which may quantify symptomatology. Laboratory studies could also be extended to psychological testing, such as neuropsychological testing, studies of learning patterns and learning disabilities, and blood level studies of medication to correlate with treatment response.

The fifth phase comprises natural history studies that attempt to answer the questions: Given the index population of patients, what happens to them over time? Can meaningful subgroups be formed based on differential outcome? The last phase involves studies of all modalities of treatment in all combinations.

The implication of this model is that children, who present with the same clinical picture of a disorder defined solely on phenomenologic grounds, may form different subgroups in terms of etiology. These subgroups of the original sample might be picked up by laboratory studies or family studies, or by differential responses to identical treatment. In 1972, I suggested this model would be quite appropriate for the study of ADD and gave some preliminary findings from the available literature suggesting that stimulant responders and non-responders might be natural groups to study. Other meaningful subgroups with regard to clinical picture might be Attention Deficit Disorder with and without Hyperactivity. Tests of the study of the utility of this latter subgrouping have just now been undertaken in a variety of studies.

With regard to physical and neurologic factors, the presence of minor physical anomalies might define a subgroup of ADD children as might the presence and type of "soft" neurologic signs. Obviously children with associated organic brain disorders, such as cerebral palsy and epilepsy, probably also form a separate group.

Family studies have suggested that there is an increased rate of ADD in close family relatives, including parents, of ADD boys, and also suggest that there may be an increased rate of the antisocial spectrum disorders: alcoholism, antisocial personality disorder, and hysteria.

There are now solid laboratory studies in the electrophysiologic area, the biochemical area, studies of blood levels, studies of attentional measures such as the continuous performance task, and others. Natural history studies have also been undertaken over the last 10 to 15 years that have been of three types: prospective studies, true retrospective studies and catch-up prospective studies. These studies suggest that, in adolescents, at least somewhere between 50–60% of probands with the disorder in childhood will continue to manifest symptomatology in adolescence. They also suggest that the disorder may predispose to certain other types of disorders in adolescents, such as severe educational retardation, antisocial personality disorder and, possibly, dysphoric syndrome.

Retrospective studies and catch-up prospective studies suggest that the disorder may persist into adult life and that when one searches for adults with the disorder one may find higher prevalence rates in females than what would be expected considering the prevalence rate of the disorder in childhood.

Finally, treatment studies have been dominated in the past years by short-term stimulant response studies. Now, newer drugs are being studied. Other types of intervention are being compared with stimulant drug treatment and being used in combination with drug treatment.

With such a burgeoning literature, it is not surprising that it is hard to keep up with major advances in the field. One of the difficulties is that each set of investigators tends to concentrate on one or two areas of this model. It is, therefore, useful to have symposia such as those under the direction of Lewis Bloomingdale, where active investigators in the field can come together and discuss some of their current findings with people who are looking at the same problem from another area.

A brief sampling of some of the papers presented at the Third High Point Hospital Symposium illustrates the interactive effect of this model and the value of this type of symposium. Sergeant, for example, from the clinical picture standpoint, has conducted a study looking at several aspects. One of the most important is the nature of the attention deficit, which is ill-defined in the DSM-III category of Attention Deficit Disorder with Hyperactivity (ADDH) and without Hyperactivity. Sergeant (Chapter 1) distinguishes between a deficit in one or more of the attentional processes (such as encoding, search decision and response organization) or deficits in attentional strategy. By comparing children who are rated as having attention and distractability problems, with and without hyperactivity, he found that the DSM-III subtypes of ADD with and without hyperactivity may be a useful subdivision. Much further work is necessary on the nature of the attentional processes that might be disordered in ADD with and without hyperactivity and it may be that these subtypes will also differ in outcome, response to treatment, prevalence rate in boys versus girls, etc., which could be investigated by other areas of this model.

Hicks and Gualtieri (Chapters 5 and 6)† looking at the differential psychopharmacology of methylphenidate on the neuropsychology of childhood hyperactivity, postulated that what might characterize ADDH is a trait of excessive variability. Central to the therapeutic effect of methylphenidate and other stimulants may be the homeostatic effect of stimulants in reducing response variability. They suggest a neuroanatomic locus of childhood hyperactivity in terms of a disorder or dysmaturation of the frontal-striatal system. Their laboratory studies, correlating blood levels with response to treatment with methylphenidate, combine two areas of this model: the laboratory study with treatment response. Their data suggest that blood level determinations of methylphenidate will not likely become part of routine clinical management because of the variability in the association between blood level and response to medication.

Huessy and Howell (Chapter 2) have made a valuable contribution to the study of ADD by their continued follow-up, of a prospective nature, of 501 second-grade students in northwestern Vermont. They were able to follow these children and interview them at the age of 21. Even when a total population sample is selected, the number of girls who meet the criteria for ADDH is relatively small. Nevertheless, it is interesting that their outcome suggests that girls may eventually present with a clinical picture of hysteria in young adult life. Hysteria is rarely if ever described in males; sociopathy, which is a relatively common outcome of ADD in males, is relatively uncommon in females. Previously, I have suggested that ADD may be a common precursor to hysteria in females and to sociopathy in males; these may be alternate forms of expression of the same underlying features in adult life, since these disorders are known to be related, from family and adoption studies. Conversion symptoms, which are unexplained pseudoneurologic symptoms, occur mostly commonly in females with hysteria and next most commonly in males with sociopathy. Huessy's data are consistent with other data, starting from the opposite end by studying adults who are presenting with ADD symptomatology and whose symptoms have been present since childhood. These studies have not only suggested high rates of a dysthymic disorder but also high rates of hysteria in the females who were identified. Family studies suggest a high rate of antisocial spectrum disorders, sociopathy and alcoholism in males, and hysteria in females. Studies of the parent of male probounds with ADDH are quite consistent with Huessy's data and with other studies suggesting that girls may be at risk for hysteria.

Quite a different result was obtained by Satterfield and his colleagues in their 8-year prospective study of delinquency in ADDH males (Chapter 17).† It was quite clear that ADDH males have much higher delinquency rates compared to a normal control group and also higher rates than 35 non-ADDH brothers of ADDH subjects. Delinquency data in the Satterfield study were based on official arrest records and not simply on what the subjects told them, which is a major advance in published outcome studies. Satterfield et al also followed 100% of the original identified group. Coupled with data they have presented elsewhere, suggesting that there may be electrophysiologic measures in childhood that distinguish those ADDH boys who eventually become seriously delinquent from those who do not, the data are quite exciting because they suggest that not only do we know that ADDH is a significant precursor for delinquency, but we may also be able to identify, early in childhood, those children who are more likely, among the total population of ADDH children, to become delinquent.

A number of presentations at the ADD-III symposium looked at the issue of treatment response in relationship to laboratory evaluation. Simeon and Ferguson (Chapter 9)† looked at treatment response not to a psychostimulant drug but to a new antidepressant drug, bupropion. This drug, the tricyclics, and ther pharmacologic effect is not well understood.

There was enough clinical improvement in 17 children with ADDH treated with bupropion to stimulate a multicenter trial. The drug seemed not only to affect hyperactivity but also anxiety symptoms, depressive symptoms, other emotional symptoms and eating disturbance. Whether bupropion will be replaced on the market is questionable at this time, but "drug dissection" studies may be used with a total population of children. In these studies the same children could be treated with methylphenidate or other psychostimulant, with imipramine or other tricyclic antidepressants, or with bupropion, for significant lengths of time to see if independent groups could be identified which respond better to one drug than they do to another, or respond well to one drug and actually get a negative response from the other. Such studies have been few and far between. However, when conducted in conjunction with biologic measures, such as biochemical measures, electrophysiologic measures, neuropsychological measures, they could go a long way in identifying potentially etiologically different subgroups of the ADDH syndrome.

Shekim and his group have been pioneers in studying responses to ADDH and its relationship to urinary and plasma levels of MHPG, the major metabolite of norepinephrine, and other biochemical abnormalities (Chapter 11)†, Their current studies revealed that ADDH children excrete lower levels of MHPG and HVA (the major metabolite of dopamine) in their urine, compared to controls. They also found that dexedrine decreased MHPG levels while increasing HVA levels. D-amphetamine was found to correct a negative correlation between HVA and MHPG in the ADDH children. There may also be an association between the disturbance in catecholamine metabolism and learning difficulties, which warrants further research and explanation. This brings us back to the clinical picture phase of my model, subdividing the original population on the basis of those with and without learning disabilities, to see if other biochemical, neuroendocrine, electrophysiologic, attentional, or other correlates could be found.

Serfontein (Chapter 12) also found that, as a group, ADDH boys excreted lower levels of MHPG, a finding largely attributable to a subgroup with very low levels of MHPG. It was found that the ADD boys with more normal baseline MHPG responded better clinically to methylphenidate and also showed a concurrent decrease in MHPG excretion after treatment, again suggesting a correlation between baseline MHPG excretion and change in MHPG excretion (the laboratory phase of my model) and increased behavioral and clinical response (the treatment phase of the model).

In summary, the papers in this book are a collection of contemporary, ongoing, cutting-edge research in the syndrome of ADDH. Interactions at symposia such as these cannot help but lead investigators who have been looking at the syndrome from one standpoint to organize their thoughts in certain others areas of the model that I have proposed, all of which are sure to increase our knowledge base and ultimately benefit the large number of children who present with this syndrome and who seem to be at risk for psychopathology later in life.

DENNIS P. CANTWELL, M.D.

1

Functional Deficits in Attentional Deficit Disorder?

JOSEPH SERGEANT

INTRODUCTION

DSM III implies a distinction between Attentional Deficit Disorder (ADD) with and without hyperactivity. Unfortunately, the definition of attention disorder rests only on behavioral observations of the child. Crucial to the distinction is the concept "attention span." Three general points will be made concerning the relation between ADD and attention span: (a) no clear distinction is made between attentional *processes* and attentional *strategies*; (b) it is unclear which of these contain the ADD dysfunction; and (c) there is no clear model of how ADD relates to controlled information processing. This chapter considers these issues and argues that the functional deficit of ADD children may lie in their deficient attentional *strategy*.

Our terms are considered in relation to the model schematically presented in Figure 1.1. Two general classes of information processing

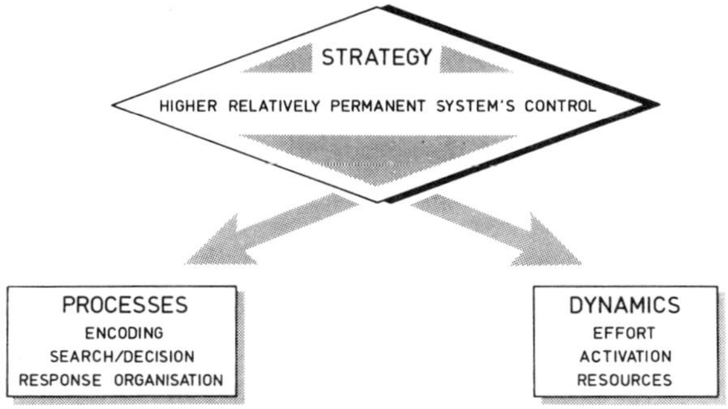

FIG. 1.1 The two classes of information processing models: *Mechanics* of processing and the *dynamics* of processing are conceived to be related to one another by a rather permanent control operation which may adjust the quality and nature of attentional functioning.

models appear in the experimental cognitive literature. The first is a model of the mechanics of processing. Here processes of attention are considered as mechanics or mechanisms. Usually, the process mechanics cited are: encoding, search/decision and response organization (Sternberg, 1969; Shiffrin and Schneider, 1977). The mechanics are structural processes usually with constant stage output and sometimes presented serially (Sternberg, 1975), sometimes in cascade (McClelland, 1979), or as semi- or completely discrete stages (Miller, 1982). A contrast to the mechanics of the processing approach is the capacity model approach to attention.

Capacity models consider limitations in human performance as due to restrictions in the quantity of energy made available to meet task demands (Kahneman, 1973). Resources are here conceived of as energetic intervening variables, rather than as the mechanics of information processing as described in the stage model (Sternberg, 1975; Sergeant and Scholten, 1983). Capacity-resource models assume that by loading the subject through task variables, such as display load or instruction set, that the quantity of resources will be increased until some limit is reached (Navon and Gopher, 1979). Since instruction set may require a speed or accuracy emphasis, resource allocation may reflect the subject's cognitive strategy (Pachella, 1974).

The concept strategy, if used too loosely, can probably be discarded as one with surplus meaning. However, if it is defined carefully and tied it to rather specific measures, it may be extremely helpful in relating previously described mechanics and dynamics of cognitive processing to one another. It is defined here as a characteristic of higher, and relatively permanent, operation of a system's control. A subject's strategy may interfere with the order and accuracy with which mechanics are run in processing. On the other hand, a subject's strategy may lead to inappropriate deployment of effort or resources in a task. A discrepancy may arise between the subject's actual state and the state required for a task (Hamilton *et al.*, 1977). Here our concern is with respect to strategy as measured in a trade-off in the quality of the subject's performance.

Separation of structural process deficits from strategy effects is no simple matter. One solution is to administer all levels of the task variable (here display load) in each of three instruction conditions: accuracy, normal, and speed (Ollman, 1977). In its simplest form, a structural model would predict that any difference in deficits observed between the hyperactives and controls would be apparent under all instruction sets. A difference in the divided attention parameters (reaction-time, slope and errors), with instruction sets between groups, would be considered as evidence of a strategy defect. Consider Figures 1.2 and 1.3. Both represent theoretical data from subjects. The first point is that discovery of a difference between ADDs and a control group, as indicated on the top panel of Figure 1.2, is not in itself evidence that ADDs have an attentional deficit. It merely

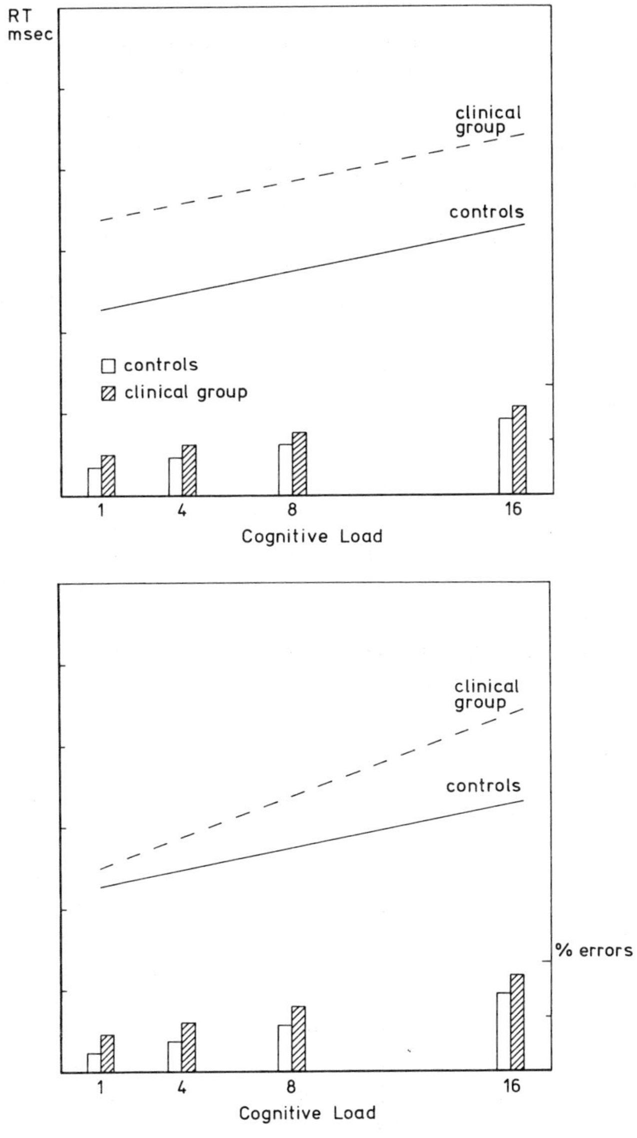

FIG. 1.2 The top panel indicates only group differences on a task. The bottom panel indicates both a group difference and interaction with the selective attention variable cognitive load. This would be evidence of a selective attention deficit in the clinical group.

indicates that controls are faster and more accurate on the task than ADDs. Evidence of an attentional defect and, specifically, at the centrally limited processes of research and decision is shown on the bottom panel of Figure 1.2. Here ADDs are not only slower and less accurate than controls but,

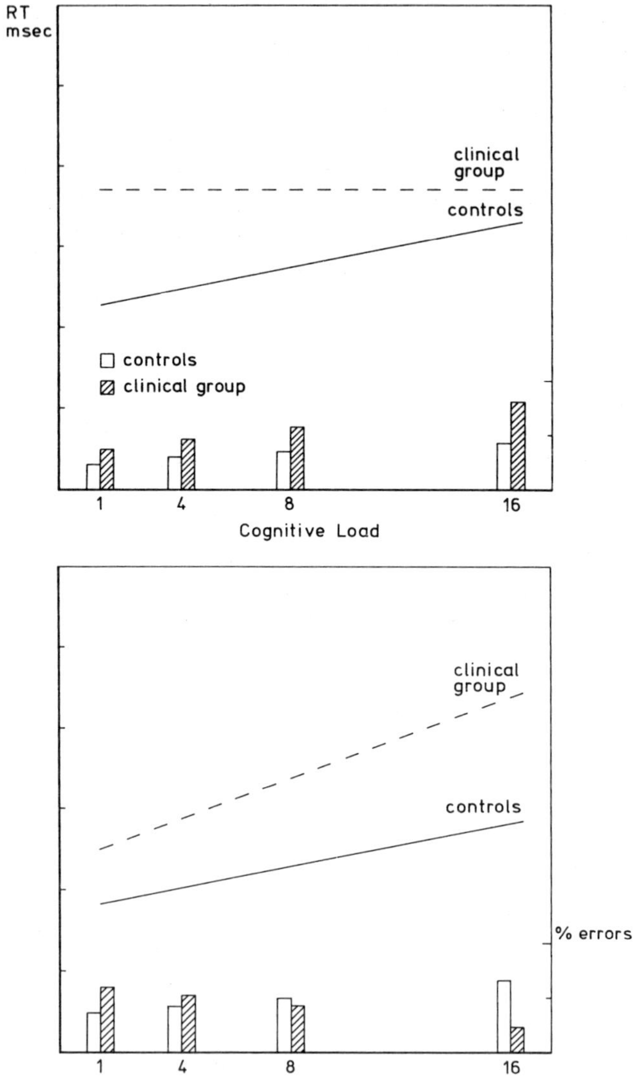

FIG. 1.3 Two examples of attentional strategy differences between groups. On the upper panel, the clinical group maintains speed of performance at the cost of accuracy. In the lower panel, the clinical group maintains accuracy at the cost of speed of performance.

as task demands increase, the speed of cognitive processing slows down more than in controls. This is, following Schneider and Shiffrin, 1977, evidence that a limitation in capacity has occurred, since capacity limitations are manifested as restrictions in the rate of the controlled processes: search and decision.

Two examples of evidence of differential strategies between ADDs and controls are given in Figure 1.3. On the upper panel, controls do not trade speed of processing for accuracy of processing as the task load increases. In other words, there is a positive correlation between the two measures of task performance. The clinical group, in contrast, meets the increasing levels of task demands by maintaining a relatively constant speed of processing, but the accuracy of processing decreases. This would lead to a negative correlation between task performance measures. On the lower panel, the clinical group now applies a strategy in which accuracy improves with load, but speed of processing increases with task demands. Is there a model which takes into consideration subjects' strategies in an attentional task?

One model, which relates the speed and accuracy of processing, the fast guess model (Yellot, 1971), proposes that strategy effects may be accounted for in the following manner: correct processing occurs when stimulus evaluation has occurred and responses are stimulus-controlled. Such processing costs time. The model predicts that correct responses are slow. Error responses occur when response initiation begins before processing is completed. Such responses are fast guesses. If the relation that errors are fast and accurate responses are slow was observed to a greater degree in hyperactives than controls, it would be a considerable empiric foundation for the clinical concept "impulsivity," which is associated with the hyperactivity cluster (Clements and Peters, 1962).

Strategy solutions to test demands have been reported to differ between hyperactives and controls in research with the Matching Familiar Figures test. Hyperactives are reported to commit more errors and to have a shorter response latency (Campbell *et al.*, 1971, 1977; Cohen *et al.*, 1972; Hopkins *et al.*, 1979). This relationship: fast processing leading to high error rates, slow processing with low error rates, is formalized in the fast guess model. Should hyperatives conform to this formal model, considerable support would be given to the notion that hyperactives are cognitively impulsive.

Evidence of strategy differences between hyperactives and controls in attentional tasks is limited, since few studies have reported both accuracy and speed in relation to task demands. The possibility of a trade-off may be seen in the insightful study by Sprague and Sleater, 1977. Here cognitive load was manipulated in relation to placebo and dosage levels. Sprague and Sleater noted large load effects on the accuracy with modest effects on the latency of performance. Considering that these authors observe a high degree of inaccuracy (between 15% and 40%), it is highly possible that trade-off between speed and accuracy was present in this experiment. Recently, Rosenthal and Allen, 1980, in a speeded-classification task, observed no difference between hyperactives and controls in the speed of processing. They noted, "the sensitivity of reaction time as a dependent variable was compromised since there were significant differences in the number of errors committed across test conditions. Consequently, trade-offs between speed and accuracy factors reduce the sensitivity of reaction time when strategy effects seem to play a role".

Consequently, this paper reports manipulation of speed and accuracy. A speed emphasis will, invariably, elicit fast but less accurate processing; whereas an accuracy set will generate slower and less error-prone processing. Should performance differences occur between hyperactives and controls as a function of instruction set, it would be important to discover whether such differences were due to a failure in processes, such as search and decision, or to resource allocation. Previous research by us has shown clear differences between hyperactives and controls on search tasks without, however, any evidence of a selective attention deficit (Sergeant and Scholten, 1983). The results given in the present paper have been fully reported elsewhere; the reader is referred to these papers for full details of method and results (Sergeant and Scholten, 1985a, b).

METHOD

Subjects

The behavioral profile for each of the three groups of boys ($N + 8$) who took part in the experiment is shown in Figure 1.4. As may be seen from the figure, the hyperactive group of children has a higher mean rating on activity and distractibility than the distractible and control children. This may be seen in a slightly different manner in Figure 1.5. In this figure the minimum, maximum, mean, 25th, and 75th percentiles are plotted for each of the three groups of boys. As can be seen from Figure 1.5, the control and distractible groups have a much lower mean and range of overactivity than the hyperactives. This was essential to show that the distractible group is not significantly different from hyperactives on distractibility ratings, but has a clear difference in this activity rating. All subjects were attending normal school; their ages ranged from 8.0 to 12.0 years.

Task Stimuli and Procedure

For those unfamiliar with the terms employed in fast processing research, it would seem profitable to give some additional information on how an attentional deficit is identified with the task variable load (as indicated previously in Figure 1.2). Load in this experiment was manipulated through requiring the subjects to process more letters displayed on a screen. In Figure 1.6 an attempt is made to represent the lowest level of load. Basically, the subject is informed to retain in memory a single letter—in the example, the letter "P." He sees four masks (stars) followed by two letters and two masks. The subject is required to respond with a

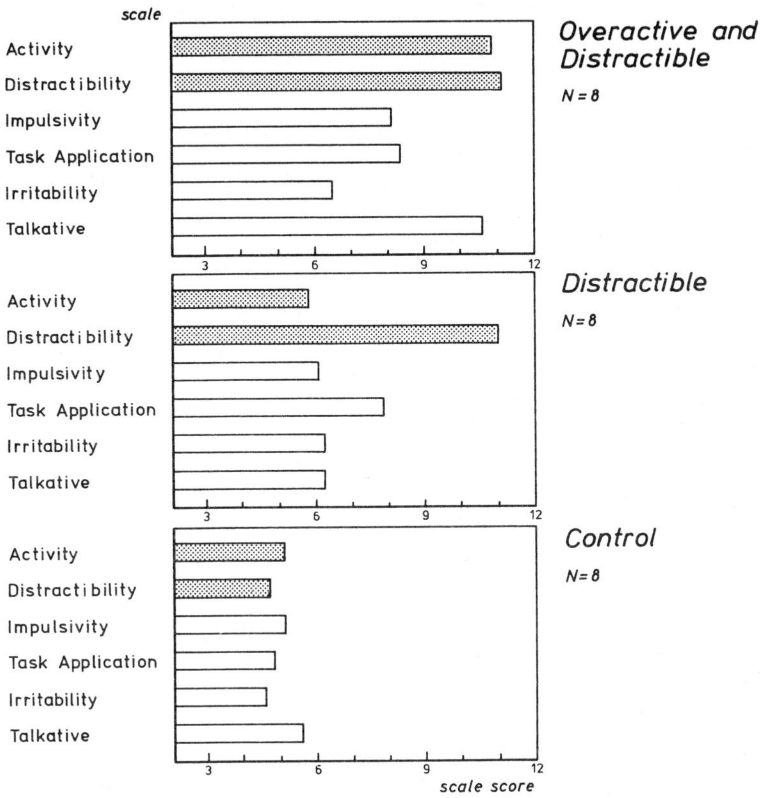

FIG. 1.4 Group profiles: criteria scales are the etched bars used to select children for group membership.

finger deflection indicating "yes" when the target is present or "no" if absent. Each trial commenced with the masks (which acted as a warning signal). The target letters employed were for display load equals two, the letter "R"; for display load equals three, "D"; and display load equals four, the letter "N." An example of display load equals four is shown in Figure 1.7. In display load four, the subject has more letters on display to process. The number of letters retained in memory as target remains one.

Before each level of load was administered, the subject received 20 practice trials. These were repeated until the subject had perfect performance.

Instruction Sets

Three instruction sets were employed in the experiment: normal, speed and accuracy.

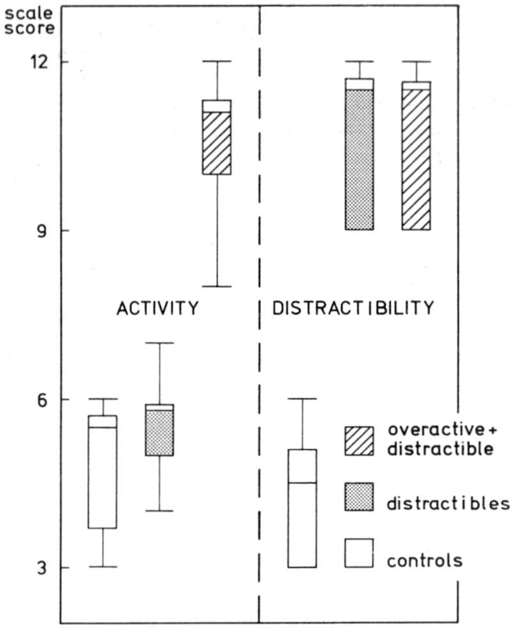

FIG. 1.5 Bar diagrams of the activity and distractibility scale scores for each group of subjects. Each bar provides the maximum and the minimum scores; the 25th and 75th percentiles; and the middle bar shows the median score.

In the normal condition, subjects were instructed to place as much emphasis on the speed of their reactions as on the accuracy of their responses.

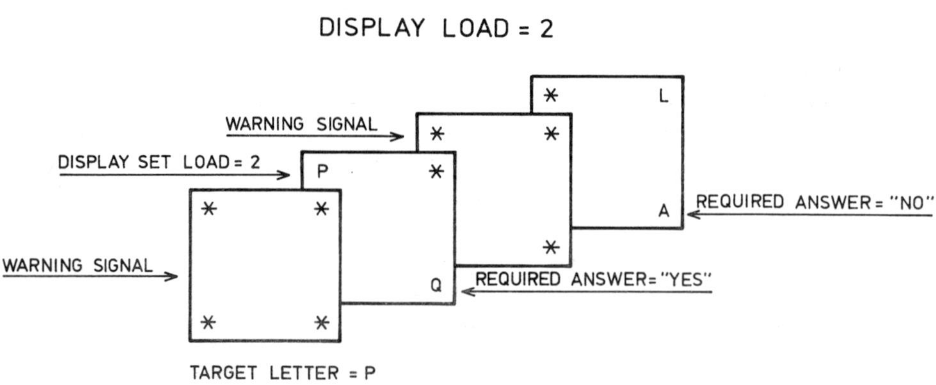

FIG. 1.6 The subject is warned by four stars of an imminent letter display. Display load is two. Memory load is one. When target is present, the subject is required to press a "yes" switch. When the target is absent, the subject is required to press a "no" switch.

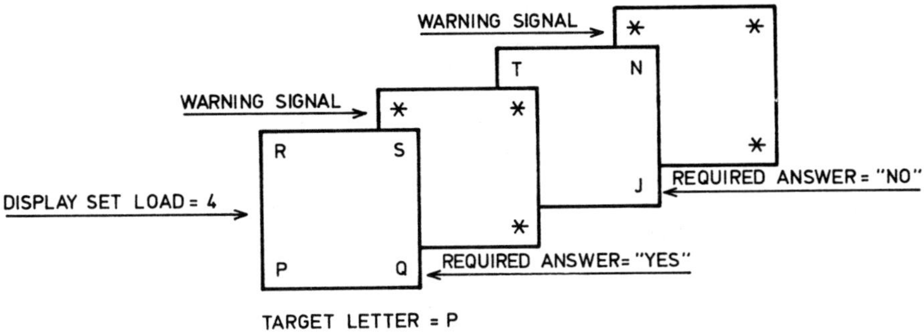

FIG. 1.7 An example of increasing the display load. Here the display load is four units. Memory load remains constant with one unit. All other arrangements in the timing and intervals between stimuli remain as when the display load was two units.

Speed instructions required that the child execute his responses as fast as possible without concern for accuracy. At each catch trial (trials where only the warning signal occurred) the experimenter exhorted the child to increase his responding, to be as fast as possible.

Accuracy required that he slow his responses to such a degree that he was confident that he would not commit an error. Speed of responses was not important, only that each response be correct.

In both accuracy and speed conditions, the child was informed that on trials in which he committed errors in the accuracy condition, or slow responses in the speed condition, he would lose 5 marbles from his sack of 15.

EXPERIMENTAL RESULTS AND DISCUSSION

The main results from this experiment were that ADDs with overactivity and without overactivity were clearly distinguishable from controls in being slower and less accurate in their cognitive processing. Despite clear evidence of the operation of selective attention demands in this experiment, neither ADDs with or without overactivity showed interactions with the task variables: search and decision. Clear instruction effects were observed in the experiment. Instruction sets interacted with selective attention demands. Instructions differentiated between both groups of ADD children and controls. (A full description of the statistical results is given in Sergeant and Scholten, 1985a).

Structural Demands

Structural task demands exerted by cognitive load were highly significant in this experiment (see top panel, Figure 1.8). As predicted by

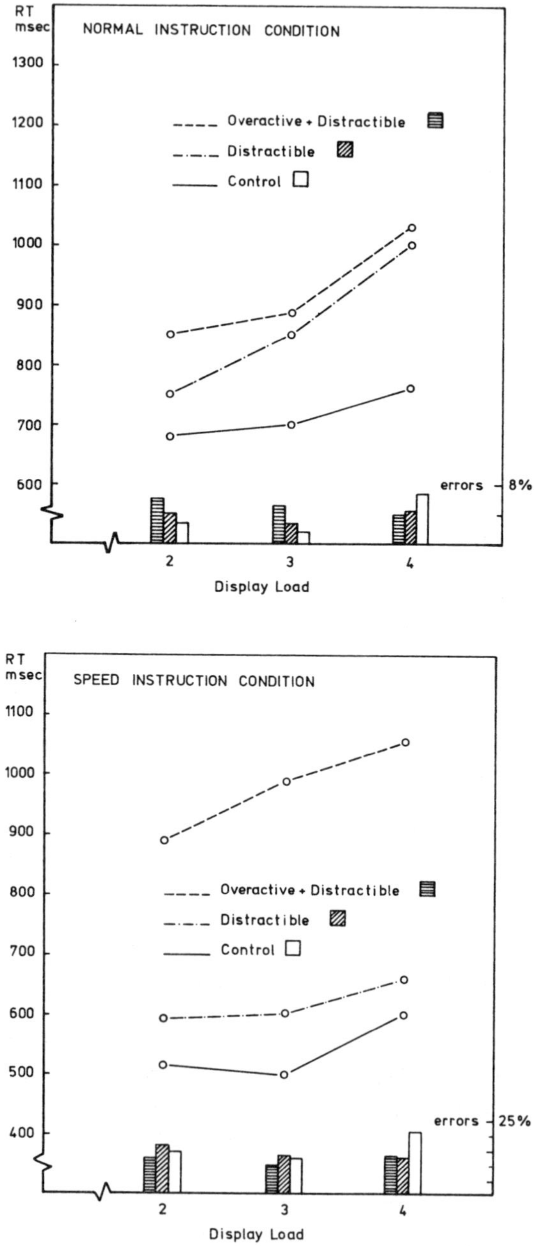

FIG. 1.8 Reaction times and errors for each subgroup in "normal" and speed set condition. In a speed set, overactive and distractible rated children fail to speed up in performance, although they increase in error rate. This is evidence of a strategic performance limitation in this group.

the model, both search and decision interacted, thus indicating controlled processing demands in the experiment ($F = 14.0$ (1,21); $p < .001$).

Group Classification and Structural Demands

All three groups of children differed in the speed of processing. However, the slower processing of the ADD subgroups was not explained by structural task demands.

Task Dynamics and Group Classification

Clear differences were required in cognitive processing through the instruction sets: speed, normal and accuracy (compare Figures 1.8 and 1.9). As may be seen from Figures 1.8 and 1.9 ADDs with overactivity perform slower than ADDs without overactivity ($F = 11.9$ (2,21); $p < .001$). In an accuracy set instruction (see Figure 1.9), both ADD groups operate slower than controls.

This study clearly indicates that although structural task variables operated and demanded selective attention, neither group of ADDs could be shown to have an attentional process deficit. The evident demands placed on all groups by the dynamic variable instruction sets, in contrast, did interact with group classification. These results suggest that ADDs are to be characterized as exhibiting an attentional strategy dysfunction.

Failure to observe evidence of a process deficit in ADDs has been reported by us earlier (Sergeant and Scholten, 1983). This has been replicated and reported (Sergeant and Scholten, 1985b). In the schema shown in Figure 1.10, a summary is provided of the structural task experiments conducted by us thus far.

The schema in Figure 1.10 suggests that with the type and range of task variables used in our series of experiments, there is little evidence of an attentional *process* deficit when divided attention demands are required. The failure to find evidence of structural deficits in ADDs, which would implicate a divided attention deficit, is consistent with a recent review by Douglas and Peters (1979). They concluded that the interpretation placed upon results by experimenters had overstated the case for an attentional deficit. The present data suggest that the loss of behavioral control, which is rated in the items of DSM III (as shown in Table 1.1), may reflect more the dynamics of behavior than the mechanics of attentional processing. This line of reasoning is supported by a recent study by Parry and Douglas, 1983. Effects of continuous and partial reinforcement were studied in hyperactive and control children in a concept identification task. It was reported that rather than an informational feedback deficit in hyperactives, a motivational factor could explain the results.

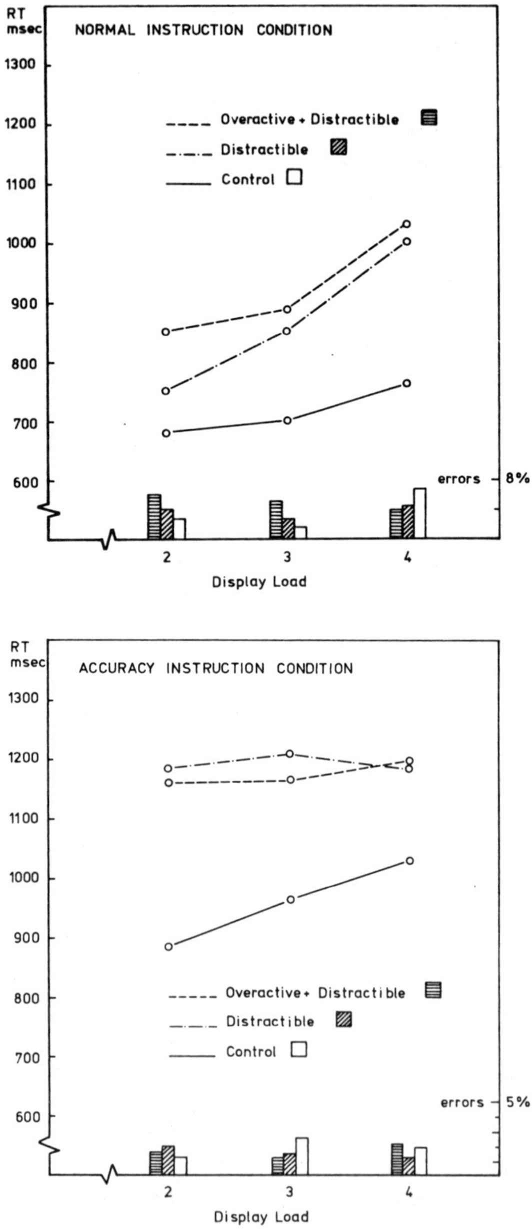

FIG. 1.9 Group performance in the "normal" and accuracy sets. Both groups of ADD children adjust their performance to ensure that the lowest load level speed of responding can meet all increases in cognitive load. This is an example of strategy differences with controls and not evidence of a selective attention deficit.

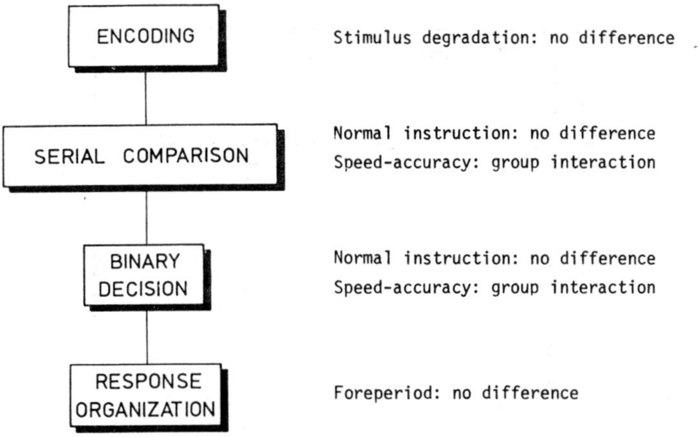

FIG. 1.10 An overview of structural and dynamic task variables in relation to ADD *with* and *without* overactivity rating.

The position adopted here is that structural deficits in ADD have not been implicated by a wide variety of task variables. The claim that ADDs suffer from a sustained attention deficit (Sykes *et al.*, 1971, 1973; Aderson *et al.*, 1973; Dykman *et al.*, 1979; Grunewald *et al.*, 1975; Klorman *et al.*, 1979; Sergeant, 1979; Sostek *et al.*, 1980; Spring *et al.*, 1973) has not always been replicated (Weingartner *et al.*, 1980). Five points should be noted concerning the above sustained attention studies.

1. Sustained attention deficit evidence is primarily from the CPT or comparable task. This task involves many processes such as encoding, working memory relations, search, decision and response organization (Sergeant, 1983). When the CPT discriminates between hyperactives and controls, which of these processes is responsible for the poor performance outcome?

2. It should be noted that the data supporting the sustained attention deficit hypothesis is primarily from analyses of error data. Such data cannot be used to discriminate between the alternatives that the product of the information chain is truly deficient in one or more of the above processes, or that the deficit is due to a change in the dynamics of processing (for example, allocated resources or effort).

3. The sustained attention deficit hypothesis encounters difficulties when, on the one hand, error data from the CPT suggested that hyperactives perform poorly over time. When latency measures are used on the same subjects, no differences between hyperactives and controls can be found in choice or serial reaction time (Sykes *et al.*, 1971). On the other hand, when time-on-task effects are measured and found to discriminate between hyperactives and controls, such effects do not interact with divided attention demands (Sergeant and Scholten, 1983).

4. Inspection of published figures in support of a sustained attention deficit seldom actually show a pattern of ADDs increasing their error rate with time-on-task. What is shown is that the ADDs maintain their performance level over time; controls, in contrast, improve their performance. This is a typical practice effect.

5. The CPT data are interpreted in terms of a vigilance deficit. That is, the sensitivity of the subject to discriminate signal from noise trials. The proponents of this hypothesis have to explain why, when additional noise is administered in the CPT, hyperactives are not differentially affected by increasing noise (Sykes *et al.*, 1971). Furthermore, when sensitivity to competing inputs is demanded in dichotic listening, hyperactives have not been differentiated from controls (Davidson and Prior, 1978; Loiselle *et al.*, 1980). In addition, the sensitivity measure has not always been reported in relation to the response bias measure, which should be theoretically independent but has been reported to be correlated in hyperactives (Sostek *et al.*, 1980).

Despite this general lack of evidence implicating a process deficit in hyperactivity, it is possible that task variables, which exert greater load upon the subject and directly influence the rate of processing, may provide the necessary interactions between task variables and group classification.

Presently, the data suggest that the strategy and the dynamics of processing, which have primarily been studied from the point of view of the Matching Familiar Figures test (Campbell *et al.*, 1971; Cohen *et al.*, 1972; Hopkins *et al.*, 1979), could better be studied in tasks requiring real-time processing.

It is concluded that, since ADDs *with* and *without* overactivity may be differentiated from one another and show interactions with the dynamics of processing, the distinction made by DSM III is a useful one.

ACKNOWLEDGMENTS

This work was partially supported by a grant from the Netherlands Organization for the Advancement of Pure Research (W.O.). The author gratefully acknowledges the assistance of L. Leertouner in drawing the figures in the chapter.

GENERAL DISCUSSION

Dr. Swanson: Your task is excellent for evaluating hyperactive children and comparing them with normal children. It provides an order of magnitude greater than the continuous performance task (CPT), which is irrelevant to salient issues in attentional dysfunctions, and is similar to the Sprague task used to study dose-response functions and different tasks with different dose-response functions.

Dr. Sergeant: If Sprague's data are plotted for placebo conditions against load, the slope is flat but errors increase with load, which we showed here. Dr. Sprague agrees that this is a strategy effect.

Dr. Swanson: That is the critical issue about task specificity in evaluating normal vs. hyperactive children. Even more important in evaluating drug response is an appropriate task such as you and Sprague used. You will probably find overdose effects on lower doses of drugs on this task than on the CPT task.

Dr. Sergeant: Evidence from the psychostimulant studies show that these drugs influence the response organization, not the central search and decision. Frowein (1981) showed that barbiturates influence the stage and amphetamines, the response organization. The response side and the search and decision side should both be manipulated, to learn how drug level influences the entire process.

Dr. Swanson: Sprague studied dose-response functions with the task and found an effect on errors, not on speed. Whether evaluating increasing speed or increasing errors, both are incorporated in one matrix.

Dr. Sergeant: It is quite a technical issue (Pachella, 1974). Information transmission is not the same as task-variable search and decision.

Dr. Hicks: Sprague gave us a set of raw data on this task, using MPD, placebo and thioridazine. Under control conditions, intrasubject correlation between latency and accuracy is highly negative. It switches to positive with Mellaril. MPD turns the correlation towards zero. In other words it stops trading speed for accuracy, confirming that it does not change the way the processes work; it changes the way they are deployed. (Cf. Gittelman-Klein *et al.*)

Dr. Sergeant: Those data really show that the activation effects of MPD specifically influence the strategy. I don't recall a response organization variable with Sprague's tasks; his variables were of the same type I used with the memory search. The bottom line is that distractables operate like controls, trading speed and accuracy in almost the same way. Under normal instructions, they tend to be fast and make errors. The extreme group shows both slow processing and very inaccurate responding. For research purposes, we are now able to distinguish between the groups in terms of processing dynamics. There must be, I believe, a higher control mechanism, partially unavailable or only temporarily available to the hyperactive. Inattention is not being measured in the sense that those children cannot do anything; they can do many things, but their control is highly limited.

Dr. Simeon: It seems you are using the concept of the function of attention deficit and distractability interchangably. You are measuring distractability as a different function from attention span; but attention is not distractability either. Children can have extremely poor attention but are not at all distractable. For example, autistic children cannot pay attention; on the other hand, they are not distractable.

Dr. Sergeant: When a child looks at our display, we find no difference between the hyperactive, the distractable, and the control group in the interval between the warning signal (that is, when the child has been commanded to attend) and the point at which the child makes his response originally. The difference starts to appear immediately after the response, until the subsequent warning signals. Then some children start to move about and look around. This is the point at which we distinguish the groups from one another (Sergeant and Scholten, 1985a). The hyperactive child looks at the display, correctly prepares his responses, but he is slow and inaccurate. Thus, he is attending, in the sense of: "I am looking at the display, doing what the experimenter told me to do," but his information processing of the data is poor. (Cf. Rapoport *et al.*, 1978.)

Dr. Pelham: No one, to my knowledge, has looked at the relationship between the parameters you describe and what others measure and define as "on task" behavior in the classroom. Your attentional characteristics may be completely different from those cognitive psychologists call attention on such tasks. What do you predict will happen to the slope differences between hyperactives and normal when controlling for error?

Dr. Sergeant: I still expect to find the answer to that; it is the whole point of the experiment. To get it, the children have to undergo about 9 hours of testing, which must be spread over sessions. One must be extremely careful about how that task is performed because it involves a very clear relationship with the child. Observers have stated: "We can distinguish the hyperactives from the controls by your behavior because you are structuring the task for the children; you are giving them instructions whereas you tell controls just to go on with it." So actually more than just processing is involved; I am structuring the child's behavior.

Dr. Pelham: Instead of thousands of trials couldn't you set a contingency? That is, tell the child his error rate is maximal and if he goes above it, he will have to do the task until he performs it at or below the maximum error?

Dr. Sergeant: You can first focus on accuracy to get the error rate right, then start working on the standard deviation. In a number of experiments standard deviation changes as a function of drug manipulation. We need to know the variance and that mean reaction time faithfully represents true processing time. If the standard deviation is greater than 10% of the mean, that is noise. There may be so many scattered points in the data that noise rather than true processing is measured.

Dr. Swanson: One task hyperactive children can do easily is a Sternberg (1975) scanning task with either 1-, 2- or 3-digit numbers. Little practice is necessary to reach a criterion in which the standard deviation is reasonable with respect to the mean. If 1 to 4 items are memorized, using 2 digit numbers, e.g., 24, 56, 15 as items, and then probe with the 2-digit number, a very similar situation is obtained. I developed and reported a model, based on normal adults, related to the prediction of error function as well as reaction times. The variation you present, combining memory and display loads, seems to be an excellent task to study some of the issues you raised.

Dr. Sergeant: We often examined event rate and how fast stimuli are presented to children. Too fast a time gives a very high error rate and slower processing. When demands for sustained attention are increased, subjects change strategies. There is some evidence for this in search tasks where operators use screens. Extreme care is needed when looking at evidence on sustained attention deficits.

Dr. Pelham: This also suggests an interesting way to start separating impulsivity from inattention, since you have the speed/accuracy trade-off. Impulsivity is the other cognitive deficit Douglas talks about.

Dr. Hechtman: We looked at some of these factors, developmentally, in children and young adults without drugs. On the matching familiar figures and imbedded figures tests, we found that as subjects grew older their reaction times increased, but not with a relative decrease in errors. In other words, they learned not to react as quickly but to process. Although your findings show they may have made more errors initially and taken longer, as the load increased their errors decreased, which meant that they did learn to process.

Dr. Sergeant: I don't think it is "either/or." I think it is "both/and." There are children whose reaction times have slowed but who still make errors, because we have internal codes—both optimal and nonoptimal—inside short-term memory. The speed of processing is the reaction time. The model predicts that with time the codes build up so that the subject, to be accurate, should work on optimally efficient codes. His accuracy may increase and he may work on even more efficient codes, but the feature of the model is the recovery time. The codes do not always remain in short-term memory in optimal character. After a certain period of time, the subject's reaction time improves but his accuracy is actually lower. Now this carries a prediction: not only is the mean reaction time slower but the type of errors made are not false alarms, they are misses. Because the target is presented so rapidly, the optimal code decays and the child no longer optimally processes targets.

REFERENCES

Andersen RP, Halcomb CG, Doyle RB: The measurement of attentional deficits. Except Child 1973; 39:534–539.

Campbell SB, Douglas VI, Morgenstern G: Cognitive styles in hyperactive children and the effect of methylphenidate. J Child Psychol Psychiat 1971; 12:55–67.

Campbell SB, Endman MW, Bernfield A: A three-year follow-up of hyperactive preschoolers into elementary school. J Child Psychol Psychiat 1977; 18:239–250.

Clements SD, Peters J: Minimal brain dysfunction in the school-aged child. Arch Gen Psychiat 1962; 2:185–197.

Cohen NJ, Weiss G, Minde K: Cognitive styles in adolescents previously diagnosed as hyperactives. J Child Psychol Psychiat 1972; 13:203–209.

Davidson EM, Prior MR: Laterality and selective attention in hyperactive children. J Abnorm Child Psychol 1978; 475–481.

Douglas VI, Peters KG: Toward a clearer definition of the attentional deficit of hyperactive children. In CA Hale and M Lewis (eds): Attention and Cognitive Development. New York, Plenum Press, 1979.

Dykman RA, Ackerman PT, Oglesby DM: Selective and sustained attention in hyperactive learning-disabled and normal boys. J Nerv Ment Dis 1979; 167:288–297.

Frowein HW: Selective effects of barbiturate and amphetamine on information processing and response execution. Acta Psychol 1981; 47:105–112.

Gittelman-Klein R, Klein DF, Katz S, Saraf K, Pallack E: Comparative effects of methylphenidate and thioridazine in hyperkinetic children. Arch Gen Psychiat 1976; 33:1217–1231.

Grunewald-Zuberbier E, Grunewald G, Rasche A: Hyperactive behavior and EEG arousal reactions in children. EEG Hyperactive Clin Neurophysiol 1975; 38:149–159.

Hamilton P, Hockey GRJ, Reyman R: The place of the concept of activation in human information processing. In S Dornic (ed): Attention and Performance 6. Hillsdale, NJ, Erlbaum 1977.

Hopkins J, Perlman T, Hechtman L, Weiss G: Cognitive style in adults originally diagnosed as hyperactives. J Child Psychol Psychiat 1979; 20:209–216.

Kahneman D: Attention and Effort, Englewood Cliffs, NJ Prentice-Hall, 1973.

Klorman R, Salzman LF, Pass HL, Borgstedt AD, Dainer KB: Effects of methylphenidate on hyperactive children's evoked response during passive and active attention. Psychophysiology 1979; 16:23–29.

Loiselle DL, Stamm JS, Maitinsky S, Whipple S: Evoked potential and behavioral signs of attentive dysfunctions in hyperactive boys. Psychophysiology 1980; 17:193–201.

McClelland JL: On the time relations of mental processes: An examination of systems of processes in cascade. Psychol Rev 1979; 86:287–330.

Miller J: Discrete versus continuous stage models of human information processing: in search of partial output. J Exp Psychol Human Percept Perf 1982; 8:273–296,

Navon D, Gopher D: On the economy of human information processing systems. Psychol Rev 1979; 86:214–255.

Ollman R: Choice reaction time and the problem of distinguishing task effects from strategy effects. In S Domic (ed): Attention and Performance VI. Hillsdale, NJ Lawrence Erlbaum Associates, 1977.

Pachella RG: The interpretation of reaction time in information-processing research. In B Kantowitz (ed): Human Information Processing: Tutorial in Performance and Recognition. Hillsdale, NJ. Erlbaum, 1974.

Parry PA, Douglas VI: Effects of reinforcement on concept identification in hyperactive children. J Abnorm Child Psychol 1983; 11:327–340.

Rapoport JL, Buchsbaum MS, Zahn TP, Weingartner H, Ludlow C, Mikkelsen EJ: Dextroamphetamine: cognitive and behavioral effects on normal pre-pubertal boys. Science 1978; 199:560–563.

Rosenthal RH, Allen TW: Intratask distractibility in hyperkinetic and nonhyperkinetic children. J Abnorm Child Psychol 1980; 8:175–187.

Schneider W, Shiffrin RM: Controlled and automatic human information processing: I. Detection, search and attention. Psychol Rev 1977; 84:1–66.

Sergeant JA: Memory search in children with a hyperactivity rating. In M Cesa-Bianchi and M Poli (eds): Aspetti Biosociali Dello Sviluppo, F Angeli, Milan, 1979, pp 223–234.

Sergeant JA, Scholten CA: Encoding, search and decision in hyperactivity. J Child Psychol Psychiat 1983; 24:49–60.

Sergeant JA, Scholten CA: On data limitations in hyperactivity. J Child Psychol Psychiat 1985a; 26:111–124.

Sergeant JA, Scholten CA: On resource strategy limitations in hyperactivity. J Child Psychol Psychiat 1985b; 26:97–109.

Shiffrin RM, Schneider W: Controlled and automatic human information processing: II. Perceptual and learning, automatic attending, and a general theory. Psychol Rev 1977; 84:127–190.

Sostek AJ, Buchsbaum MS, Rapoport JL: Effects of amphetamine on vigilance performance in normal and hyperactive children. J. Abnorm Child Psychol 1980; 8:491–500.

Spring C, Greenberg L, Scott J, Hopwood J: Reaction time and effect of Ritalin on children with learning problems. Percept Mot Skills 1973; 36:75–82.

Sprague RL, Sleator EK: Methylphenidate in hyperkinetic children: differences in dose effects on learning and social behavior. In WG Kostger (ed): Attention and Performance II. Amsterdam, Elsevier/North-Holland, 1977.

Sternberg S: The discovery of processing stages: extensions of Donders' method. Acta Psychologica 1969; 30:276–315.

Sternberg S: Memory Scanning: new findings and current controversies. QJ Exp Psychol 1975; 27:1–32.

Sykes DH, Douglas VI, Weiss G, Minde KK: Attention in hyperactive children and the effect of methylphenidate (Ritalin). J Child Psychol Psychiat 1971; 12:129–139.

Sykes DH, Douglas VI, Morgenstern G: Sustained attention in hyperactive children. J Child Psychol Psychiat 1973; 14:213–220.

Weingartner H, Rapoport JL, Buchsbaum MS, Bunney WE, Ebert MH, Mikkelsen EJ, Caine ED: Cognitive processes in normal and hyperactive children and their response to amphetamine treatment. J Abnorm Psychol 1980; 89:25–37.

Yellott JI: Correcting for fast guessing and the speed-accuracy trade-off in choice reaction time. J Math Psychol 1971; 8:159–199.

2

The Behaviors Associated with ADD Followed from Age Seven to Twenty-one: Differences Between Males and Females

HANS R. HUESSY AND DAVID C. HOWELL

We have been involved in a prospective study of 501 second-grade students in Northwestern Vermont. The students represented all of those in the second grade at the schools studied. The study began in 1965 and the subjects were subsequently interviewed at age 21. Details of this study have been reported in previous volumes of this series. Here we report on a reanalysis of our data when separated by sex.

The data for boys and girls combined showed:

1. Their scores on a teacher questionnaire were distributed along a standard distribution curve. High scores indicate behaviors commonly associated with hyperkinesis.
2. Children with one high score were more like those who never had a high score than like those with two or more high scores: i.e., one high score had little significance but two high scores, at least one year apart, had strong predictive power.
3. Children with two or more high scores accounted for most of the academic and social problems.
4. Children with consistently low scores were remarkably free of problems.
5. Thirteen percent of the population were identified as "at-risk": they did not warrant a DSM-III diagnosis of attention deficit disorder, but had behaviors associated with that disorder. The 13% statistic was based on follow-up results.
6. In a separate outgrowth of this study, it was also shown that 45% of male alcoholics had childhood behaviors similar to the 13% at-risk group. In another study the authors have documented that ADD frequently does not disappear in adolescence.

TABLE 2.1 *Children identified as "hyperkinetic" in previous studies by scores above 80th percentile*

Study No.	Grade[a]	Children (N)	Boys (N)	Boys (%	Girls (N)	Girls (%)
1 (1966)	2	64	44	69	20	31
2 (1968)	4	66	49	74	17	26
3 (1969)	5	63	51	81	12	19

[a] Refers to grade in which most of children studied were enrolled.

Reproduced with permission from Huessy HR, Cohen AH: Vulnerability of hyperkinetic (MBD) child to subsequent serious psychopathology: a controlled 7-year follow-up. In Anthony, Koupernik and Chiland (eds.): The Child in His Family, vol. iv. Yearbook of the International Association for Child Psychiatry and Allied Professions, John Wiley, New York, 1983.

The literature has consistently shown that boys develop ADD problems at a much higher rate than do girls. Clinically, the disorder seems to present differently and run a different course in females. For this reason the data were separated by sex. In most of their recent reports the authors separated out those individuals who scored above the 80th percentile two or more times comparing them to all of the remaining subjects. This comparison produced more clearcut results for the total population. (Previously, all subjects with one high score or more were placed in a group separate from the rest.) Our more recent method, however, produced such a small number of females that to obtain data for adult females, subjects were separated, using the original criterion of one or more scores above the 80th percentile as the cutoff.

Are high scores in boys and girls of equivalent significance? We found that boys get high scores primarily because of behavioral problems, while girls got them for educational problems. We have known for years that many ADD girls will daydream rather than move about in class. Often, serious problems arise only in early adolescence, usually around authority issues.

The percentage of girls among the children identified by our questionnaire dropped from 31% to 19% between the second and fifth grades (see Table 2.1). Table 2.2 lists the 14 questions that distinguished high scorers from normal subjects in the total population.

Table 2.3 presents the four questions that distinguished girls with one or more high scores from those who never had a high score. Nine of the 14 questions that distinguished high scoring boys were not helpful in distinguishing high scoring girls.

Some adult ADD males become sociopaths, a diagnosis seldom applied to females. Some of the ADD girls become histrionic personalities or hysterics, a diagnosis seldom applied to males. This may be an example of a differential effect of culture. With a different symptom pattern in elementary school and a different pattern of symptoms in adulthood, obviously boys and girls must be studied separately, with independently developed screening devices. Only then can the prevalence and natural history of this condition in females become evident.

Many adolescent and adult females with ADD temperaments respond to the usual anti-ADD medications. Most were not identified as problem

TABLE 2.2 *Fourteen questions that distinguished high scorers from normal subjects*

	Sex	Normal (0 or once)	ADD (2 +)	Significance (*p*)	Never (0)	ADD (1 +)	Significance (*p*)
Completed high school	M	86%	54%	0.01	90%	63%	0.01
	F	87%	89%	ns	89%	79%	ns
Education beyond high school	M	39%	20%	0.05	43%	21%	0.01
	F	41%	11%	ns	45%	11%	0.01
College prep course	M	33%	7%	0.01	39%	8%	0.01
	F	37%	11%	ns	40%	15%	0.05
Reading problems	M	28%	54%	0.01	24%	48%	0.01
	F	16%	56%	0.01	14%	39%	0.01
Suspended	M	34%	58%	0.01	31%	53%	0.01
	F	14%	0%	ns	15%	4%	ns
Employed as laborer	M	35%	68%	0.01	35%	64%	0.01
(if employed)	F	29%	25%	ns	27%	36%	ns
Four or more FT jobs	M	23%	48%	0.01	21%	40%	0.01
	F	20%	20%	ns	20%	22%	ns
"Not accident prone"	M	74%	54%	0.05	74%	61%	ns
	F	74%	44%	ns	74%	61%	ns
Injured in fight	M	24%	44%	0.01	24%	36%	ns
	F	4%	0%	ns	4%	4%	ns
Rejected for enlistment	M	10%	23%	0.05	7%	22%	0.01
	F	6%	0%	ns	5%	8%	ns
Recent police trouble	M	20%	42%	0.01	20%	32%	0.01
	F	10%	22%	ns	9%	14%	ns
Ever arrested	M	16%	38%	0.01	15%	30%	0.01
	F	4%	11%	ns	4%	7%	ns
Smokes marijuana 1/day +	M	15%	32%	0.05	14%	27%	0.05
	F	4%	11%	ns	2%	14%	0.01
Parents sought help for them for	M	11%	34%	0.01	9%	25%	0.01
behavioral or learning problem	F	12%	11%	ns	12%	11%	ns

TABLE 2.3 *Questions distinguishing high scoring girls from those without high scores*

	Sex	Normal (0 or once)	ADD (2 +)	Significance (*p*)	Never (0)	ADD (1 +)	Significance (*p*)
Education beyond high school	M	39%	20%	0.05	43%	21%	0.01
	F	41%	11%	ns	45%	11%	0.01
College prep course	M	33%	7%	0.01	39%	8%	0.01
	F	37%	11%	ns	40%	15%	0.01
Reading problems	M	28%	54%	0.01	24%	48%	0.01
	F	16%	56%	0.01	14%	39%	0.01
Smokes marijuana 1/day+	M	15%	32%	0.05	14%	27%	0.05
	F	4%	11%	ns	2%	14%	0.01

patients until early adolescence or later. Some were considered a bit self-centered, but only became problems when endless arguments about how late they could stay out, or other similar issues arose. Others gave a history of no major problems until late adolescence, when, for some days premenstrually, they would engage in impulsive behavior and be emotionally overreactive. During the next three weeks they would try to patch up the problems they had created. But things would snowball; they could not patch things up before their next episode of impulsive behavior came along. Controlling premenstrual fluid retention commonly controlled their symptoms completely. The ADD, residual type patient did not require medication other than diuretics premenstrually.

Adolescent girls presenting with suicidal gestures in emergency rooms often have long histories of emotional overreactivity and respond to small doses of the tricyclic antidepressants. These patients are frequently misdiagnosed as primary depressions and given antidepressant doses of the tricyclics. Often they experience unpleasant side effects and do not return for further treatment. The appropriate dose (much smaller) of the same medication might give them better self-control and real choices in their responses. Unfortunately for many, they are already cut off from their more "straight" peers and may not show any motivation to change. Finding a way to identify them at an earlier age might improve our chance for successful treatment and the prevention of more serious pathology. Others drop out of school, become illegitimately pregnant, or become involved in prostitution. They live in the moment, do not plan, overreact, and their problems escalate. They have produced a high percentage of infants available for adoption, resulting in a high rate of ADD among adoptees, as documented by Deutsch *et al.* (1982). In a study at an adolescent unit in a state psychiatric hospital, preliminary data show an unexpectedly high rate of adoptees among the patients, another indicator of this fact.

A study from San Antonio, Texas, indicates that the 5% of the population with low DPH (dopamine beta hydroxylase) are overrepresented in adolescent units of mental hospitals and are the most antisocial and difficult to treat when they have ADD, needing two types of medication before any benefit is achieved, usually an anti-ADD and an antipsychotic medication. Would their childhood behavioral patterns be distinguishable on our questionnaire?

A recent study of mitral valve prolapse found a prevalence of 8% in a general population and an association, especially in women, with panic disorders which, on the basis of drug response, may be related to ADD.

These are examples of overlapping groups. With 13% of all children at risk for ADD-related problems, they are likely to be represented in most major groupings of adult psychopathology.

Data from NIMH-sponsored prevalence studies (Regier *et al.*, 1984) in adult populations stress the importance of early diagnosis of ADD. The

TABLE 2.4 *ADD identified in children and adults*

Male (percentage)	Female (percentage)	Related disorders
Children		
13.0	2.0	
Adults		
4.3	1.2	Alcohol abuse
0.1	0.2	Phobias
2.8	5.8	Obsessions
2.8	4.7	Dysthymia
2.2	0.2	Antisocial
12.2	12.1	

Without major mental illness, there are 12% adult pathology in both sexes. Only 2% of females were identified during childhood, vs, 13% of males.

data presented in Table 2.4 represent the total of all diagnoses related to ADD either through epidemiologic studies or through similar therapeutic drug responses. Although the totals for these disorders are the same for men and women, the at-risk population in childhood for females could not be identified by our current data.

ADD-related adult psychopathology may occur with equal frequency in the two sexes. This makes adequate early recognition in women even more important. One ADD child may become alcoholic, another develop an explosive personality, and a third, hysteria. Panic disorder, anxiety states, phobias, some insomnias, explosive personality, many alcoholics, sociopaths, hysterics and affectively responsive depressives all have been reported to respond to small doses of tricyclics, suggesting they all share some common factor. Family studies of any of these disorders in isolation have become meaningless, since they may present differing manifestations of a common denominator. The data given in Table 2.5 exemplify that which can be found in clinical studies when the ubiquity of adult ADD is considered.

Adult depressives who met DSM III criteria and responded dramatically in less than three days to tricyclics were matched with depressives who showed the usual response pattern. As can be seen, the two patient groups differed in their personal and in their family histories. It is likely that the depressive and alcoholic relatives of the two groups, although roughly equal in numbers, may represent very different disorders. We must look for the ADD pattern in all studies of psychopathology, as many adult syndromes may represent secondary defensiive patterns of ADD children to cope with the underlying deficit.

In studies of spontaneously hypertensive and hyperkinetic rats, Dr. Edith Hendley of the University of Vermont failed to separate completely these two traits. In the hyperkinetic rat studies the biochemical pathology was located in the nucleus accumbens (Myers *et al.*, 1980).

The findings in our genetically hyperkinetic rats show that a minute amount of amphetamine, introduced directly into the nucleus accumbens,

TABLE 2.5 *Summary of Cohen's results on adults with depression and aggression*

	Unipolar depression plus aggression	Unipolar depression alone	$p \leqslant$
Males	5	5	
Females	7	7	
Mean age (yrs)	29.8	30.2	
Family history			
Violence-aggression	7/12 (58.3%)	0/12 (0%)	0.01
Poor school performance	6/12 (50.0%)	1/12 (8.3%)	0.05
Hyperkinetic relatives	4/12 (33.3%)	0/12 (0%)	0.05
Depression	7/12 (58.3%)	7/12 (58.3%)	—
Homosexual, antisocial, eccentric	4/12 (33.3%)	2/12 (16.7%)	—
Alcohol abuse	9/12 (75%)	6/12 (50%)	—
Psychoses ("nervous breakdown")	2/12 (16.7%)	3/12 (25%)	—
Childhood history			
Hyperkinetic as child	0/12 (0%)	0/12 (0%)	—
Inability to sit still, fighting, poor concentration, dropout, failure	11/12 (91.7%)	0/12 (0%)	0.005
Symptoms-signs in mental status			
Hyperactive	11/12 (91.7%)	0/12 (0%)	0.005
Distractible	11/12 (91.7%)	5/12 (41.7%)	0.025
Impulsive	12/12 (100%)	1/12 (8.3%)	0.005
Temper-aggression	12/12 (100%)	0/12 (0%)	0.005
Antisocial	7/12 (58.3%)	1/12 (8.3%)	0.025
Alcohol abuse	10/12 (83.3%)	4/12 (33.3%)	0.025
Mood swings, depression	12/12 (100%)	12/12 (100%)	—
Insomnia (0–2 hr)	8/12 (66.7%)	3/12 (25%)	0.05
Amitriptyline HCl (100–250 mg)	8/10 (80%)	8/12 (66.7%)	—
Imipramine HCl (40–200 mg)	3/10 (30%)	8/12 (66.7%)	ns
Less than 7 days for remission of sx's	10/10 (100%)	0%*	0.005
Sleep induction and initial depression on medicine	8/10 (80%)	1/12 (8.3%)	0.025
BPRS decrease	19.6 (1 week)	16.9 (6 weeks)	

p Values based on Fischer exact probability test.

* Mean, 5.0 weeks; range 1–8 weeks; one patient had no benefit.

Reproduced with permission from Huessy HR, Cohen SM, Blair CL, Rood P: Clinical explorations in adult minimal brain dysfunction. In Bellak (ed.): Psychiatric Aspects of Minimal Brain Dysfunction in Adults. New York, Grune and Stratton, 1979, p 25.

replicates the effects of a much larger oral or intravenous dose. Norepinephrine uptake was higher than that in controls, whereas dopamine uptake was lower. This may help to explain some of the variability in drug response.

Perhaps physiologic instability is part of all or some ADD, and physiologic tests for overreactivity may hold some promise. It has been suggested that an increased percentage of ADD problems occur today because, until the advent of antibiotics, the ADD child may have been the one who had unusually high fevers and a differentially higher mortality rate from infectious diseases. Many of the most seriously ill cases may have been children who, in the past, died.

The social cost of ADD-related pathology is immense. Close to one-half of alcoholics, a high percentage of delinquents and adult criminals, early school dropouts, many illegitimate pregnancies (complicated by the disaster of these girls trying to raise their babies alone while supported by welfare), a sizeable part of the problem of child abuse, job instability and family instability may be consequences of ADD. Any amelioration, however slight, of these problems would have tremendous human cost benefits. At Spring Lake Ranch, a therapeutic community for chronic mental patients, I have been able to diagnose and treat a number of schizophrenics, who also suffered from ADD, residual type, and did much better when tricyclic treatment for the latter condition was added, a good example of the overlapping of types of pathology mentioned above. I would suggest that studies of successful adult ADDs would provide more information about factors that allow these individuals to become successful rather than problem adults. More rational and perhaps more successful intervention, based on these study results, might be possible. Early identification of females and identifying factors common to a successful outcome should be a priority. For many of these children, symptoms can be minimized with drugs that seem to be reasonably safe. Their poor self-image, lack of self-confidence, impaired education and poor social networks, which are the results of many years of ADD, are often impossible to overcome later. It is very discouraging when an adult ADD responds well to medication, but his/her poor self-image and negative past seem to make progress impossible. Methods are needed to identify the young female at risk, to encourage early control of symptoms in both sexes, and to study the successful adult ADD to find better methods of intervention and support strategies, and the sexes must be studied independently.

GENERAL DISCUSSION

Dr. Shekim: I missed your point on the early differences between boys and girls.

Dr. Huessy: Questionnaires designed to identify ADD do not differentiate boys from girls. My assumption is that adult female pathology must have its antecedents, too, and is probably identifiable; we do not know how to identify it in childhood.

Dr. Shekim: Adult ADD is more prevalent in females than in males, while it is the reverse in childhood ADD.

Dr. Huessy: That may be due to distortions in adult diagnoses.

Dr. Quay: If instead of talking about top 20% scores, you spoke about children who are less intelligent, are of lower socioeconomic status, and are more aggressive, would your results be the same?

Dr. Huessy: Although Vermont is considered a poor state when classified by socioeconomic status, surprisingly a greater number of patients were not in the lower SES. Of our original group, no patient had been on welfare, so that SES could not have been important. IQ varied—the higher the ADD score the lower the IQ tended to be, although differences were not great. The problem is that of the chicken or the egg. When we controlled for IQ, the findings persisted.

Dr. Quay: As I see it, relating negative adult outcomes to the results of your questionnaire are a problem, without some kind of statistical control for those variables known to be significant, such as SES, IQ and the tendency to behave aggressively.

Dr. Huessy: The children with high scores on our questionnaire seemed to have most of the negative outcomes. Aggression by itself (a few questions dealt with aggression) was not a better predicter alone, it did not have the accuracy of the total questionnaire. Neither aggression nor IQ accounted for much of the predictive power.

Dr. Quay: You said that as the adults remembered themselves as children, they did not report they were hyperactive. In the interview on mental status, they had a high incidence of impulsivity and hyperactivity. Is this correct?

Dr. Huessy: We designed the questionnaire and gave it to adults who had gone through our study. We sent it to some who had high and some who had low scores and they were amazingly accurate when returned. On this basis we gave the questionnaire to adult alcoholics, and obtained some data that make us think it might have some validity.

Dr. Ferguson: Paul Wender's data, some of your other work, and reports by Ralph Tarter, have provided a lot of data indicating that if alcoholics are asked what they were like as children, many report behavior suggestive of hyperactivity. Do you know of any longitudinal psychiatric studies with data showing that in families where alcohol is a problem, childhood hyperactivity is a discriminating factor for subsequent alcohol problems?

Dr. Huessy: Twenty-two years old may be too early for that probability. People who admit to calling themselves alcoholics are usually older.

Dr. Hechtman: In follow-up studies we found that alcoholism tends to be a cumulative risk factor. If the hyperactive child grows up in a negative family, and has a low IQ (they might also have learning disabilities as well), all of these risks factors, additively, make it more likely that their outcomes would be negative, one of which would be alcoholism. Having an alcoholic in the family and being hyperactive may or may not, in and of itself, be sufficient. If the family is also in a low socioeconomic class and the child has a somewhat lower IQ, then chances are increased.

Dr. Huessy: I'd suggest studies of adopted children who present with these kinds of problems to a fairly severe degree. Here you can have a high socioeconomic status, well-functioning families and eliminate such complications. A perfectly healthy family may adopt a genetically loaded boy who goes in the wrong direction, regardless of what the adoptive parents do.

REFERENCES

Deutsch CK, Swanson JM, Gruell JH, Cantwell DP, Weinberg F, Baren M: Overrepresentation of adoptees in children with the Attention Deficit Disorder. Behav Genet 1982; 12:231–238.

Myers MM, Whittemore SR, Hendley ED: Forebrain catecholamine mechanisms in the spontaneously hypertensive rat. In E Usdin, R Kvetnansky and IJ Kopin (eds): Catecholamines and Stress: Recent Advances. Elsevier, North Holland, 1980.

Howell DC, Huessy HR: A fifteen year follow-up of a behavioral history of Attention Deficit Disorder. Pediatrics 1985; 76:185–190.

Huessy HR, Cohen AH: Hyperkinetic behaviors and learning disabilities followed over seven years. Pediatrics 1976 57:4–10.

Huessy HR, Preis K: Hyperactive children at risk. In MJ Cohen (ed.): Drugs and the Special Child. New York: Gardner Press 1978; pp 129–187.

Huessy HR, Cohen SM, Blair CL, Rood P: Clinical explorations in adult Minimal Brain Dysfunction: A developmental approach. In L Bellak (ed.): Psychiatric Aspects of Minimal Brain Dysfunction in Adults. New York: Grune and Stratton 1979; pp 19–36.

Huessy HR, Howell DC: The relationship between adult alcoholism and childhood behavior disorders. Psychiatric Journal of the University of Ottawa 1985; 10:114–119.

Regier DA, Myers JK, Kramer M, Robins LN, Blazer DG, Hough RL, Eaton W, Locke B: The NIMH epidemiologic catchment area program: historical context, major objectives and study population characteristics. Arch Gen Psychiat 1984; 41:934–941.

3

The Combination of Behavior Therapy and Methylphenidate in the Treatment of Attention Deficit Disorders: a Therapy Outcome Study

WILLIAM E. PELHAM,
ROBERT W. SCHNEDLER, MARY E. BENDER,
DAVID E. NILSSON, JAMES MILLER, MARY SUE BUDROW,
MARILYN RONNEI, CAROL PALUCHOWSKI,
AND DAVID A. MARKS

Although psychostimulant medication has been widely used for many years, current findings have suggested that as the sole treatment for attention deficit disorder (ADD), it is an inadequate form of intervention. Problems surrounding the use of high doses include adverse physiologic, cognitive, and social effects (Mattes and Gittelman, 1983; Sprague and Sleator, 1977; Pelham, 1983; Pelham and Bender, 1982; Swanson and Kinsbourne, 1979). When low doses are administered to avoid these possible difficulties, most of the children treated fail to improve to the point at which no further intervention is needed (e.g., Sleator and von Neumann, 1974). Perhaps the major limitation regarding medication is that, without exception, studies in which children were treated with stimulants for periods up to 5 years have failed to provide evidence that the drugs improve the long-term prognosis of ADD (Charles and Schain, 1981; Riddle and Rapoport, 1976; Satterfield *et al.*, 1982; Weiss *et al.*, 1975).

These limitations of psychostimulant medication have led to the interest in behavior therapy in the treatment of ADD. Behavior therapy is not used as widely as psychostimulant medication (Bosco and Robins, 1980), but it has generated more research than any other alternative to medication. Although early studies suggested that behavior therapy was as effective as psychostimulant medication (Ayllon *et al.*, 1975; O'Leary *et al.*, 1976; O'Leary and Pelham, 1978; Pelham, 1977), more recent studies have cast doubt on the sufficiency of behavior interventions for ADD. A substantial proportion of treated children fail to show improvement, and many of those who do improve fail to reach a normal range of functioning (Abikoff and Gittelman, 1984). Some studies even failed to find that behavior therapy had a significant effect on ADD children (Loney and Milich, 1983). Finally, the effectiveness of behavior intervention depends on the competence and willingness of teachers and parents to implement the treatment (Pelham and Murphy, 1986). If the responsible adults are unable or unwilling to conduct programs as taught by behavior therapists, behavior interventions will not be effective.

Given these limitations of both behavior and pharmacologic interventions, our research has focused for several years on whether combining these treatment modalities might lead to more effective intervention than either alone has proved to be. Specifically, we have been interested in whether psychostimulant medication can be used to enhance the effects of standard, clinical, behavior interventions. Several individual cases suggested that this was a possible outcome. Two children treated by O'Leary and Pelham (1978) and the child treated by Pelham (1977), when withdrawn from psychostimulant medication and treated with behavior therapy, exhibited such severely disruptive classroom behavior that medication had to be reinstated. With the concurrent application of behavior therapy and methylphenidate (MPD), however, all 3 children showed improvement.

Another study (Pelham *et al.*, 1980), provided clinical behavioral intervention (parent and teacher meetings in which training in contingency management techniques was provided) to 9 hyperactive children. In addition, three double-blind, 3-week medication probes were conducted in which placebo, 0.25 mg/kg MPD, and 0.75 mg/kg MPD were each administered for 1 week. The first medication probe occurred before behavior therapy began, and the second and third probes began after 3 and 13 weeks of behavior therapy, respectively. Results revealed that most children showed maximal improvement during MPD conditions of the final medication probe, suggesting that the drug enhanced the effects of lengthy behavior intervention, and that the combined intervention was more effective than MPD alone.

The results of this study contradict those reported by Gittelman *et al.* (1980), who found that an 8-week, combined behavior and MPD treatment program was not more effective than MPD alone. Their study, however, employed a dose of MPD comparable to twice the higher of the two doses used by Pelham *et al.* (1980). During the final medication probe of our study, the effect of the lower dose of MPH was as great as that of the higher. This finding suggests that the addition of a low dose of MPD might enhance behavior intervention at the same time that it avoids the adverse side effects associated with a higher dose of the drug. Furthermore, the incremental value of the low dose was apparent only after 13 weeks of behavior therapy, suggesting that behavior interventions longer than the 8-week treatment used by Gittelman *et al.* may be necessary for maximal combined treatment effects.

In addition to the incremental value of MPD for behavior therapy, behavior interventions clearly need to expand to include peer problems. Most ADD children have serious problems with peer relationships, and if uncorrected, these problems may be predictive of a long-term disturbance (Milich and Landau, 1982; Pelham and Bender, 1982; Pelham and Bender, 1982; Pelham and Milich, 1984). Behavior and pharmacologic interventions, when used alone, have not been effective in improving disturbed peer relations (Pelham and Bender, 1982; Pelham and Milich, 1984). One study conducted in a laboratory setting showed that neither a reward program alone, nor a social skills training program alone, had a beneficial effect on observed social interactions between hyperactive and confederate children, but the combination of the two did improve social interactions (Pelham and Bender, 1982). Similar results from a single playground observation and a brief training program have recently been reported (Hinshaw *et al.*, in press). These studies suggest that an extensive social skills training program might be of incremental benefit to a clinical behavior intervention program for ADD children.

These considerations led to the current investigation. The adjunctive effects of MPD and social skills training were evaluated for children receiving a 5-month course of clinical behavior therapy. In addition, several different control groups were included to assess the effects of clinical behavior therapy.

METHODS

Subjects

Thirty-two children referred from local schools participated in the study. Twenty-two of the children, 19 boys and 3 girls, participated in the behavior therapy portion of the study. These children all met the DSM III criteria for Attention Deficit Disorders with Hyperactivity (ADD-H) and were, therefore, so diagnosed by the first author. They all exhibited problems both at home and at school. All had IQs above 85 and none had evidence of organic brain damage. All of these children received referral or pretreatment ratings above 15 on the Abbreviated Conners Teacher Rating Scale (ACTRS) (Conners, 1969; Werry *et al.*, 1975). Their mean pretreatment ACTRS rating was 19.3 ($SD = 4.2$). Most of these children also had referral or pretreatment mother ratings above 15 on the Abbreviated Conners Parent Rating Scale (ACPRS) (Goyette *et al.*, 1978). The mean ACPRS mother rating was 19.0 ($SD = 5.7$). The 4 children who did not reach a score of 15 had scores of 12, 10 (both girls), 13, and 14. In all four cases, mother ratings on the Aggressive-Conduct factor of the

Connors Parent Symptom Questionnaire (Conners, 1969) confirmed extreme behavior problems in the home setting. The 22 children in the behavior therapy groups ranged in age from 5 to 9 years (median age, 7) and were in grades ranging from kindergarten to fourth grade.

Ten other children, 9 boys and 1 girl, referred from the same schools and also diagnosed as ADD-H, participated in a social-skills-training, contrast-treatment group. These children ranged in age from 6 to 10 years (median, 8) and all had a score above 15 on the ACTRS ($\bar{X} = 20.1$; $SD = 5.1$). Parent ratings were not available for these children, but home problems were consistently reported.

An additional group of deviant children was made up of 2 from the contrast treatment group and 2 who had been referred for, and accepted into the program but whose parents declined treatment. Permission was obtained to gather observational data on these children. Although admittedly a very small group, they constituted a no-treatment control in the sense that they did not receive behavior therapy and their observational data were so analyzed. As the other treated children, these 4 boys were diagnosed as ADD-H and had ACTRS ratings above 15 ($\bar{X} = 23$; $SD = 2.3$).

Finally, for each ADD child, his or her teacher selected several normal classmate controls of the same sex who did not exhibit behavior or learning problems. These children served as a normal comparison control group for the observational measures. One of the several children named in each classroom was designated as the primary normal control, and teacher ratings were gathered on them. The mean ACTRS rating for these children was 1.7 ($SD = 1.7$).

Procedure

Design

Treated subjects were divided into five groups. Four groups received standard, clinical, behavior therapy (parent and teacher training in contingency management), as well as one or both of two adjunctive treatments. These four groups were formed by crossing drug condition (MPD vs. placebo) with social skills training condition (training or no training) to yield four adjunctive treatment combinations that were provided in addition to the clinical behavior therapy. The 22 first children who had been referred and accepted into the study were divided into quartets based on age and then randomly assigned within quartets to one of these four groups: (a) behavior therapy, MPD, social skills training (BT-MPD-SS; $N = 5$); (b) behavior therapy, placebo, social skills training (BT-PL-SS; $N = 6$); (c) behavior therapy, MPD, no social skills training (BT-MPH-No SS; $N = 6$); and (d) behavior therapy, placebo, no social skills training (BT-PL-No SS; $N = 5$). A fifth group of 10 children was recruited slightly later than the first 22 subjects. These 10 children were all assigned to a contrast-treatment, control group, who received social-skills training only.

Dependent measures

A complete set of dependent measures was available on the children assigned to the behavior therapy groups. Pre- and post-treatment measures were gathered on the ACTRS and ACPRS, Wide Range Achievement Text (WRAT) (Jastak *et al.*, 1978), positive and negative peer nominations (Pelham and Bender, 1982), and direct observations of classroom behavior (Mash and McElwee, 1976). In addition to these pre- and post-treatment ratings, teachers made ACTRS ratings midway through treatment on children who were in the behavior therapy groups. Only peer nominations and ACTRS were available for children in the social skills training contrast-treatment groups, and only classroom observations for the small, ADD-H, no-treatment control group.

Before and 3 weeks after treatment had terminated, sociograms of the positive and negative nomination type were administered in the children's classrooms. In individual sessions with a tester, children first pointed to and named all of their classmates on a class picture. Then each child was asked to point to, in the picture, and name three children whom he or she liked and three children whom he or she did not like. The total number of negative nominations received by each child served as the dependent measure.

Before and from 1 to 4 weeks following treatment, each child was observed in his or her classroom. The observational code used was Mash and McElee's (1976) adaptation of Patterson's (1976) code. This code includes 42 behavioral categories that describe social interactions that occur between children and adults. Six additional categories were added that were deemed necessary to detect behaviors that were likely to be shown by ADD children. A pool of 17 observers were trained to use the code and do the observations. Training followed the procedures recommended by Mash and McElwee (1976) and included practice with videotapes and in-classroom settings. Observers were trained to a criterion of 70% agreement on tapes and in classroom practice prior to gathering data in the study.

Each treatment child was scheduled for 10 pre-treatment and 10 post-treatment observations over 4-week periods before and following treatment. The mean number of observations actually made was 8.9 ($SD = 1.9$) pre-treatment and 8.8 ($SD = 1.9$) post-treatment. Observations were made at times of the day, almost always in the morning, when the children's classes were engaged in academic activities. The observations were usually made at times when the target child was to be engaged in independent seatwork, although some observations occurred when the target child was engaged in a group teaching activity.

Each observation lasted for a sufficient time for the observer to complete six observation forms. Each form represented 6 consecutive minutes of observation divided into 5-second blocks. On half of the observational days only the ADD child was observed. On the other half of the days, the observer alternated between the ADD child and his or her normal comparison control. The primary, normal comparison child was observed unless absent, in which case one of the other teacher-designated normal controls was observed.

The dependent measure derived from the observations consisted of a higher-order category selected a priori. Negative behavior (a sum of interrupting an activity, destruction, noncompliance, negative physical action, high rate, and self-stimulation) was a rating of inappropriate behaviors that characterize ADD children. Scores on this category reflect the proportion of intervals that any of the subordinate categories were recorded out of the total number of intervals observed each day for an individual child. Each child's scores were averaged across all pre- and post-treatment observations to provide the scores used in the analysis of observational data.

Behavior therapy

The behavior intervention was conducted over a period of 5 months. Seven therapist (two PhD level and five MA level) worked with the families and teachers. All therapists had experience with behavior techniques, five of them having had extensive experience. Each therapist's cases were distributed as much as possible across adjunctive treatment groups. Therapy involved a standard approach to clinical behavior therapy, focused on teacher and parent training in contingency management, as described extensively previously (O'Leary *et al.*, 1976; O'Leary and Pelham, 1978; Pelham, 1978; 1982; Pelham *et al.*, 1980). After an initial assessment of the children's problem behaviors, therapists met in separate weekly individual sessions with the children's parents and teachers.

Parent training began with assigned readings, *Families* (Patterson, 1976) and discussion of the principles of social learning. Together, the parents and therapists devised contingency management programs to modify the children's specific problem behaviors. Procedures used included: praising appropriate behavior, ignoring minor inappropriate behavior, punishing with time out or loss of privileges for more serious instances of inappropriate behavior, and the implementation of Premack contingencies and incentive systems. Reward programs were used in all cases to provide consequences for good daily reports from school and, in most cases, to reward changes in home behavior. Individualized rewards included:

special family activities, extra time before bed, allowances, television time, and long-range goals such as a new bike or watch.

All of the teachers were, to some extent, familiar with behavior approaches to classroom management. After brief discussions of the principles of social learning, teachers and therapists worked together to devise programs to deal with each child's specific problem behaviors. In all cases, a daily report card was instituted. Three to five target behaviors were evaluated daily and the child took the report home, where predetermined rewards were provided for having met the specified criteria. In all cases, completion of assigned classwork and getting along well with other children were target behaviors. Not disrupting the classroom or disturbing the teacher was frequently a target. Daily reports were changed over the course of therapy, as was necessary. In addition to daily reports, teachers used a variety of procedures in the classroom, including praising and ignoring, time out, and Premack contingencies (e.g., work completed before recess or free time upon class completion). In all cases, successive approximations to the final goals were carefully shaped.

Towards the end of the intervention, parent and teacher sessions were held only biweekly, or even less often. Several of the final parent meetings were held in small groups. The mean number of parent sessions was 9.7 ($SD = 2.4$; range = 4 to 13), and the mean number of teacher sessions was 10.3 ($SD = 2.1$; range = 7 to 14). Therapists met as a group weekly and discussed cases and procedures in order to maximize treatment standardization. Therapy began in January, immediately following the pre-treatment assessment period, during which ratings and observations were made, and it was completed in May, approximately 1 week before post-treatment observations began and 3 weeks before other post-treatment dependent measures were gathered.

Social skills training

Children who received social skills training met in eight Saturday morning group sessions held at a local school. They met in groups of 10 to 12 children with four or five trainers (one graduate student and three or four undergraduates) for 3 hours each Saturday. Sessions were designed to provide instruction in aspects of positive social interaction, practice in displaying appropriate social behavior in a peer group context, and rewards for appropriate peer interactions. In 10- to 20-minute, small-group, teaching sessions, instruction, modeling, and role-playing techniques were used to teach and demonstrate appropriate social behavior. The concepts addressed in these small-group sessions included communication, participation, cooperation, and validation-support (Oden and Asher, 1977). Each brief teaching session was followed by a 30-minutes period when the children played a game as a group (e.g., red light, green light; red rover, red rover). During the game period, trainers used praise to reinforce children playing appropriately. In addition, children could earn points for displaying the social skills they had been taught in the instructional periods. They received feedback, regarding their points during brief feedback sessions at the end of each game period. These points could be exchanged at the end of each Saturday session for tangible reinforcers (small toys, candy, gum).

Over the eight sessions, children were taught to evaluate their own behavior following a procedure described by O'Leary *et al.* (1975). The feedback sessions following games began with the trainer prompting the children to evaluate their behavior and tell why they had lost or gained points. Children were asked to predict how many points they were going to receive. During the first four sessions, the trainers then gave the children feedback and told them how many points they had earned. During the fifth and sixth sessions, children's predictions had to come within one point of matching the trainer's evaluation to receive their points. During the last 2 weeks of social skills training, the children's self evaluations had to match exactly their trainers' ratings to receive points.

Medications

When behavior therapy began for children who received it, either 0.3 mg/kg MPD or placebo administration began (on school days only) for children in the behavior therapy groups. In absolute amounts, the mean dose was 8.5 mg MPD per administration (17 mg/day for those who received two doses per day). Per dose, 3 children received 10 mg; 4 took 8.75 mg; 3 took 7.5 mg; and 1 received 6.25 mg. Most children took MPD with both breakfast and lunch, but children who were in kindergarten and attended school for only half a day took only one morning pill. All participants in the study and all project staff except the director were blind regarding medication condition.

MPD was encapsulated, and matching placebo was prepared by a consulting pharmacist. Vials of capsules were given to parents or school personnel responsible for administering medication. Parents and school personnel kept daily records of medication administration, and these records were given to therapists weekly. The records revealed that one child failed to receive medication at home and at school on a regular basis and that all other children received their medication regularly. After 10 to 12 weeks of medication, the exact length depending on the child's school holiday schedule, the noon pill was discontinued for those children receiving two per day. The every-morning administration was continued for 3 or 4 weeks, again depending on school holiday schedules, after which point all pills were discontinued and behavior therapy ended.

RESULTS

One child who was in a behavior therapy group moved before post-treatment assessment. In addition, the child in the MPD group who took his medication irregularly both at home and at school was not included in any analyses because he could not be assigned to a medication group. These omissions left 20 children who received behavior therapy.

Data analysis included both analyses of variance to test for group changes as well as examination of individual data. Each child's change from pre- to post-treatment on each measure was assigned to one of three categories. Based on pre-treatment means on each measure, a 20% reduction or better was defined as improvement. Any child whose score on a measure decreased by at least 20% of the group mean was said to be improved on that variable. Any change less than a 20% improvement, but also less than a 20% increase on a measure was classified as "no change." Finally, any child whose post-treatment score was 20% or more above his pre-treatment score was classified as having become worse over the treatment period. In addition to examination of individual improvement, whether each child was within a normal functioning range, defined as within one-half standard deviation of normative means, on each post-treatment measure was noted.

Multivariate analysis

A 2 (medication) × 2 (social-skills training) × 2 (pre-post) multivariate analysis of variance was performed on the parent and teacher ACTRS rating, the negative peer nominations, and the classroom observation data from the 20 children in the behavior therapy groups. This MANOVA revealed a significant effect of pre-post, $F(4,13) = 9.37$, $p < 0.005$, but no other significant effects. In other words, there was no overall significant effect of either adjunctive treatment, but there was a significant effect of the behavior treatment (pre-post) collapsed across levels of adjunctive treatments. Following this MANOVA, in subsequent 2 × 2 × 2 univariate analyses of variance, only the pre-post effects were analyzed. The means and standard deviations, averaged across adjunctive treatments for children who received behavior therapy, are presented in Table 3.1 for all dependent measures. In addition, means and standard deviations for contrast treatment, no treatment, and normal comparison children are presented on the relevant dependent measures.

Parent ratings

The univariate ANOVA conducted on ACPRS scores showed a significant effect of pre-post, $F(1,16) = 6.3$, $p < 0.05$, reflecting lowered

TABLE 3.1 *Means and standard deviations on dependent measures*

Group	Dependent measure: Ratings[a] Parent	Ratings[a] Teacher	Negative nominations	Negative behaviors
Behavior therapy				
Pre-treatment	18.4 (5.7)	18.9 (4.0)	9.33 (4.4)	0.157 (0.076)
Post-treatment	13.5 (5.7)	12.1 (5.6)	7.35 (4.3)	0.107 (0.068)
Social skills Training only				
Pre-treatment	—	20.1 (5.1)	9.5 (3.5)	—
Post-treatment	—	16.6 (6.0)	10.9 (5.9)	—
No treatment				
Control				
Pre-treatment	—	22.8 (2.3)	—	0.105 (0.033)
Post-treatment	—	—	—	0.130 (0.057)
Normal classroom Comparison				
Pre-treatment	—	1.7 (1.7)	—	0.070 (0.044)
Post-treatment	—	—	—	0.057 (0.041)

[a] Parent and teacher ratings were made on the Abbreviated Conners Scales (Goyette *et al.*, 1978). Negative nominations are the number of negative nominations children received from peers on their classroom sociograms. Negative behavior is the proportion of observed intervals in which interruptions, destruction, noncompliance, aggression, high rate, or self-stimulation were coded during classroom observations.

scores with treatment. Forty-five percent of the children were rated by their parents as improved, compared to 45% who were rated as unchanged and 10% as worse. These percentages did not vary as a function of adjunctive treatment group. Three of the 20 children received post-treatment ACPRS ratings within one-half *SD* of the ACPRS population mean (Goyette *et al.*, 1978).

Teacher ratings

The univariate ANOVA performed on the ACTRS ratings for the children in the four behavior therapy groups revealed a significant effect of pre-post, $F(1,16) = 34.2$, $p < 0.001$, reflecting lowered scores with treatment. Eighty percent of the children in these groups improved on the ACTRS; 15% showed no change, and 5% were rated by their teacher as worse. These percentages did not vary as a function of medication condition or social-skills training. No children obtained scores at post-treatment that placed them within the range of scores obtained by the normal comparison children rated by their teachers, although 6 treated children had post-treatment ACTRS ratings that placed them within one-half *SD* of the population mean for the ACTRS (Goyette *et al.*, 1978).

A separate, correlated t test computed on the ACTRS scores for the social skills-training, contrast-treatment group revealed a nonsignificant trend toward improvement (0.10, $p < 0.20$). Forty percent of the children in this group improved, 40% showed no change, and 20% became worse. None of the children in this group obtained scores on the ACTRS within the range of the normal comparison children noted above.

A planned comparison was made of the post-treatment ratings for the children who received behavior therapy and the children in the social skills training, contrast-treatment group. The mean of the behavior therapy groups was significantly lower than that of the social-skills-only group, $t(28) = 2.0$, $p < 0.05$.

Another planned comparison was computed on the midtreatment ACTRS scores of the children in the behavior therapy groups who received MPD or placebo to determine whether their teachers viewed those who received medication as, relatively, more improved than those who received placebo, while the children were still receiving medication. This comparison revealed that children who were receiving MPD had significantly lower ACTRS scores ($\bar{X} = 6.5$, $SD = 2.9$) than children in the placebo group, ($\bar{X} = 12.7$, $SD = 6.8$); $t(17) = 2.54$, $p < .025$. Of the children in the MPD group, 80% showed greatly improved teacher rating at midtreatment on medication and a worsening of the rating at post-treatment, following MPD withdrawal. Eight of the 10 children in the MPD group received midtreatment (on medication) ACTRS ratings within one-half SD of the population mean, compared to 3 of the 10 children in the placebo group.

Peer nominations

The univariate ANOVA conducted on the negative nominations from the peer nomination measures for the children in the four behavior therapy groups revealed a significant effect of pre-post, $F(1,16) = 7.94$, $p < 0.025$, reflecting lowered scores with treatment. Examination of individual data showed that 55% of the children receiving behavior therapy improved in the number of negative nominations, 35% did not change, and 10% became worse. These percentages did not differ as a function of medication or social-skills training condition. The mean negative nominations in the classrooms of the target children were all below 3.0. Five children in the behavior therapy groups were within one-half *SD* of their class means at post-treatment (3 of them had similarly low scores at pretreatment). Seven children in these groups were more than 1 *SD* above their class means at post-treatment, while 8 additional children were more than 2 *SD* above their class means.

In comparison, children in the social skills training, contrast-treatment group showed a nonsignificant increase from their pre-treatment mean of 9.5 ($SD = 3.5$) to their post-treatment mean of 10.9 ($SD = 5.9$). Two of the 10 children in this group improved in negative nominations, 2 remained the same and 6 became worse. Both children who improved moved within one-half *SD* of their class means, although one had been within that range prior to treatment. Two of these children had post-treatment nomination scores that placed them more than 2 *SD* above class means.

A planned comparison of the post-treatment nominations for the behavior therapy and social skills training only groups revealed that the children who had received behavior therapy obtained significantly fewer nominations than did those who received social skills training only, $t(28) = 1.7$, $p < 0.05$.

Classroom observations

Reliability was checked throughout the study by having two observers observe the same child simultaneously. Reliability was calculated on a conservative, point-to-point basis, and it averaged (percentage agreements divided by percentage agreements plus disagreements) 77.2% ($SD = 10.7$; range 62% to 94%).

As in the other comparable analyses, the univariate ANOVA performed on the classroom observations of negative behavior for the children in the behavior therapy groups revealed a significant effect of pre-post, $F(1,16) = 12.0$, $p < 0.005$, reflecting lowered scores with treatment. A planned comparison contrasted the pre-post change for treated children, with the pre-post change for the 4 untreated ADD controls, and revealed a significant effect, $F(1,19) = 5.0$, $p < 0.05$. As the means in Table 3.1 show, the average negative behavior score for the 4 untreated children increased over time, in comparison to the improvement shown by the treated children. The groups were not significantly different at post-treatment, however.

A second analysis performed on the observational data involved a comparison between the classroom behavior of children treated with behavior therapy and their normal classroom controls. This 2 (group) × 2 (pre-post) ANOVA revealed a significant effect of group, $F(1,41) = 25.4$, $p < 0.0001$, and a significant group by pre-post interaction, $F(1,41) = 4.4$, $p < 0.05$. As the means in Table 3.1 show, the treated children's negative behavior scores were far above their comparison controls at pretreatment. Their negative behavior improved substantially with treatment, but the final mean level was still significantly above that of normal classmate controls at post-treatment.

Examination of individual data showed that 60% of the ADD children treated with behavior therapy improved on the observation measure, while 25% showed no change (2 of the 5 children in this group were within the normal range at pre-treatment and could not improve further), while 15% exhibited worsened behavior at post- compared to pre-treatment. Sixty percent of the ADD children obtained scores of 0.08 or below on the post-treatment observations, a score that places them within one-half *SD* of the mean for their normal classmate controls. In comparison, 1 of the 4 untreated children became worse over time, and 3 remained the same. One of these 4 children was within the normal range at both pre-treatment and post-treatment.

Achievement tests

WRAT scores were available on 17 children in the behavior therapy groups. Because social skills training was not expected to affect this measure, only medication condition was evaluated. Pre-post correlated t tests were conducted separately for the two medication groups on each WRAT subtest. The mean gains in reading, spelling, and arithmetic for the MPD group were 0.83 year ($SD = 0.59$), 0.72 year ($SD = 0.44$), and 0.45 year ($SD = 0.47$), respectively. These gains were significant at p levels of 0.005, 0.001, and 0.025, respectively ($df = 8$). Corresponding gains for the placebo group were 1.03 ($SD = 0.93$), 0.29 ($SD = 0.72$), and .28 ($SD = 40$). The placebo gains in reading and arithmetic were significant ($df = 7$) at $p < 0.01$ and 0.05, respectively, while the gain in spelling was nonsignificant ($t = 1.2$). t tests comparing the MPD and placebo gains on each subtest revealed no significant differences. The expected WRAT gain over the treatment period is 0.5 year. Collapsed across achievement subtests, 8 of the 9 children in the MPD group and 4 of the 8 in the placebo group met or exceeded the expected gain of 0.5 year.

DISCUSSION

The results from this investigation can be summarized in the following points:

1. In comparison to the contrast-treatment and no-treatment groups, and relative to their normal classmate controls, the ADD children who received standard, clinical, behavior therapy showed statistically and clinically significant improvement on all measures.

2. There were no significant pre-post effects of either adjunctive treatment. Neither concurrent social skills training nor concurrent MPD, nor their combination, significantly facilitated the degree of pre-post improvement shown with the clinical behavior intervention.

3. While medication was being administered, children who received MPD concurrently with behavior therapy were rated by their teachers as 50% better than those children who were receiving concurrent placebo. This effect did not last when medication was discontinued at post treatment.

4. There was a nonsignificant trend for children who received medication to show greater achievement gains than those who received placebo. Both groups made gains at or near the expected rates on most WRAT subtests.

5. There were large individual differences in response to behavior therapy, with from 45% to 80% of the children showing improvement, depending on the measure examined.

6. Very few ADD children obtained post-treatment scores on the dependent measures that were within a "normal" range of functioning. This was especially true with regard to the negative nominations they received from peers.

The study adds to the growing body of literature demonstrating that clinical behavior therapy is an effective treatment for ADD. The children's teachers, parents, and peers, as well as objective observers, perceived them as improved over the course of the 5-month intervention. Their improvement occurred in classroom behavior, peer relations, and academic achievement. The changes made in the behavior therapy groups are especially salient when compared to the worsening behavior shown on classroom observations and peer ratings for the contrast- and no-treatment groups. This demonstration of a beneficial effect for behavior therapy suggests that those professionals who find that behavior therapy is ineffective with ADD children have used less intensive or extensive treatment than is necessary to ameliorate ADD-H.

At the same time, these findings show more clearly that behavior therapy is not a sufficient or maximally effective treatment for the average ADD child. Although a large percentage of treated children, 80%, improved on ACTRS ratings, perhaps the most common measure of improvement in studies such as these, many fewer children showed improvement on the observation (60%) and peer ratings (55%) measures. Only 4 of the 20 children improved on all four dependent measures, and only 9 of the 20 improved on all three school measures.

Further, although 60% of the treated children moved into a normal range of functioning on the observation measures, very few of them did when teacher ratings and peer nominations were considered. Only 2 of the 20 children who received behavior therapy were within the normal range of functioning on all dependent measures at post-treatment. Especially disconcerting is the distribution of post-treatment negative nominations for the treated children. Three-quarters of the children who received behavior therapy were more than a standard deviation above their class means at post-treatment, and half of these were 2 *SD* above their means. Given the presumed predictive importance of negative peer ratings (Milich and Landau, 1982), this is a critical dependent measure, although it is the one domain in which behavior therapy appeared to have the smallest impact.

This failure is somewhat surprising, since both of our adjunctive treatments were expected to affect peer relations. Our results suggest that single-session analogue studies that show effective behavior treatments on peer interactions and provide evidence for incremental benefit from medication or social skills training should be taken with a grain of salt (e.g., Hinshaw *et al.*, in press; Pelham and Bender, 1982). At the least, a more intensive or different intervention than the one we employed appears necessary to have a major impact on peer relations. Results from a recent single-subject study suggest that peer ratings might be improved while a behaviorally treated ADD child is taking stimulant medication (Atkins *et al.*, 1984). Had sociograms been administered at midtreatment, similar beneficial effects of MPD might have been obtained. If that had been the case, however, these results show that any derived benefits disappeared within a month after the medication was discontinued.

The fact that 0.3 mg/kg MPH enhanced teacher ratings during treatment but had no lasting effect when medication was withdrawn, is at the same time heartening and disappointing. We had hoped that concurrent MPD would enhance the maintenance of whatever learning takes place when a child's behavior is modified in a behavior program. This result was not obtained. However, it is clear that concurrent administration of 0.3 mg/kg MPD and behavior therapy maximizes improvement on teacher ratings. The mean midtreatment teacher rating for the behavior therapy groups receiving MPD was 6.9, quite a low rating, and 80% of the medicated children obtained scores in this range.

A comparison of our results in this regard and those reported by Gittelman *et al.* (1980) is noteworthy. Although our MPD dose was approximately half of that used by Gittelman *et al.* (1980), the improvement in teacher ratings, the midtreatment ratings, and the final levels obtained on the teacher ratings were similar across the two studies. This suggests that maximized improvement in teacher ratings can be obtained with a combined treatment that includes a considerably lower dose of MPD than Gittelman used. In addition, the final teacher ratings reveal that our behavior intervention and Gittelman's were similarly effective. This is not surprising, as both behavior treatments were developed from O'Learys' laboratory. One difference between the studies is that significant effects of the behavior intervention were obtained on the classroom observations in our study. Gittelman's failure to find improvement with behavior intervention on classroom observations may result from the fact that her intervention was relatively briefer (8 weeks vs. 5 months).

Other differences in the results of the two studies are difficult to evaluate because of design differences. As noted above, for example, the behavior intervention was considerably longer in our study, while it did not include a medication-alone group; the post-treatment measures were taken following medication withdrawal in this study, as opposed to during medication administration in Gittelman *et al.*; and the dose of MPD that Gittelman employed was twice what we used. Had it been feasible, gathering of sociometric and observation data at midtreatment in this study would have provided information comparable to the post-treatment data reported by Gittelman, *et al.*

One final point that can be made, regarding our study and Gittelman's, is that our results suggest that Gittelman's findings of the superiority of medication and the lack of need for behavior therapy apply only as long as the children continue to take medication. When medication is withdrawn, children who have not received a long regimen of behavior therapy will presumably behave much less appropriately than those who have. Consideration of the relative merits of the separate and combined interventions needs to be made with this issue in mind. Whether medication can be withdrawn, in such a way that its incremental value will not be lost, is an important question that warrants future research.

The results of the achievement test are difficult to evaluate without an appropriate control group. Our findings that MPD tended to facilitate achievement is similar to that reported by Satterfield *et al.* (1979), who also used a multimodal intervention and a comparable dose of MPD. That study and this one are the first to have measured achievement gains with the low doses of MPD that are presumed to maximize cognitive improvement (Sprague and Sleator, 1977). Although it is tempting to conclude that a combination of this dose of MPD and a structured behavior intervention might facilitate long-term achievement gains in treated children, the lack of a control group in both this and the Satterfield studies makes such a conclusion premature. Whether stimulant medication affects academic achievement is a controversial issue that has not yet been resolved and additional research is needed (see Barkley and Cunningham, 1978; Gadow, 1983; Pelham, 1983; Pelham *et al.*, 1985; Sprague and Berger, 1980).

The importance of utilizing multiple measures of response to treatment is highlighted by our findings (see also Atkins *et al.*, 1984). Improvement varied greatly, depending on the measure examined, with the most commonly used classroom measure, the ACTRS, yielding evidence of improvement for a much higher percentage of subjects than the more objective observations and negative nominations. Similarly, the teacher ratings for the social skills training, contrast treatment group showed a trend towards improved behavior at the same time as the children's peer ratings worsened. Teacher ratings may overestimate the number of children who actually improve, yielding an overly optimistic picture of a treatment's effectiveness. This result emphasizes the need for a contrast-treatment group if teacher ratings are employed as dependent measures (Loney and Milich, 1978). At the same time, the relatively high levels of the post-treatment teacher ratings agree with the peer nominations, suggesting that the teachers are clearly aware that the children continue to have serious problems.

In summary, behavior therapy had a significant, clinical impact on ADD children's behaviors in several domains of functioning. Nonetheless, the children remained seriously disturbed on most measures following a 5-month, multimodal intervention. Behavior interventions apparently need to be more intensive and to continue for longer periods of time than that evaluated in this study before lasting improvement that approximates normal behavior is obtained (Pelham and Murphy, 1986). MPD appears to be a potentially powerful adjunct to behavior interventions, but its incremental value should not be expected to last beyond the time it is administered. Finally, combined interventions that will have a major effect on the abysmal peer relations that characterize ADD children need to be developed.

ACKNOWLEDGMENTS

This research was conducted while the authors were faculty members and students in the Department of Psychology at Washington State University, Pullman, WA, and was supported by a Biomedical Sciences grant from the state of Washington. We are indebted to the Pullman, WA; Clarkston, WA; Lewiston, ID; and Moscow, ID, schools for permission to coduct the study, as well as to all the teachers and administrators whose collaboration made the study possible. We also thank Alvin Frostad, pediatric consultant, and Sid Pierson, pharmaceutical consultant, for their cooperation. Portions of this paper were presented at the annual meeting of the Association for the Advancement of Behavior Therapy, San Francisco, CA, December 1979.

GENERAL DISCUSSION

Dr. Hunt: How does the Satterfield *et al.* (1979) study of behavior modification combined with medication relate to the Sprague and Sleator, 1977 article in *Science* showing that higher doses of stimulants impair paired-associate learning in ADDH. Some follow-up studies by others gave different results.

Dr. Satterfield: In our continued study we gave 0.3 mg/kg MPD in two divided doses. We never found it necessary to go as high as the 0.7 mg/kg dose used in the Sprague study. In fact, we feel this high dose is contraindicated if MPD is used in combination with other forms of treatment.

Dr. Pelham: The midtreatment Conners rating we obtained was probably very close to what Gittelman *et al.* (1980) reported as negative results. In their combined treatment regimen, they used twice as much medication but much less family involvement than either our or the Satterfields' study.

Dr. Huessy: Birch and Demb, in 1959 postulated that children with ADD lack the ability to respond to conditioning. Maybe medication should be given first, and if, without additional help, family and child get along fairly well, leave them alone. If more help is needed, then introduce secondary therapy. Asking parents to become therapists may cause serious role conflicts, I question the use of Ritalin in these studies because it is a short-acting drug and responses to it vary widely. There is no known standard dose.

Dr. Satterfield: Dr. Huessy's comment about the use of Ritalin is very interesting. I have used this drug successfully without the problems he ran into.

Dr. Pelham: In a just completed single subject case study, we compared 7.5 mg (0.3 mg/kg) of Ritalin twice a day with SR 20 (20 mg slow-release MPD) and with 42 mg (1.8 mg/kg) of pemoline. We found that the 7.5 mg, twice a day dose of Ritalin provided the greatest improvement in behavior. The other two drugs increased variability tremendously. I have seen other cases that showed just the opposite, that is one dose of pemoline in the morning was much better than two doses of Ritalin during the day. The only way to study treatment is by single-subject analysis. This is a very expensive method but we are trying to make it a practical one.

Dr. Thivierge: Could you describe briefly the specific behavior modication program? How much time was required per week and exactly what was done?

Dr. Pelham: We asked parents to back up our daily report card by offering the child rewards each day (e.g., free or special time with the parent, or a later bedtime), depending on how the child behaved at school, plus a special weekend activity in return for a good performance that week. In addition, as punishment parents and teachers are taught to use time out instead of a spanking. Some times we set up point systems at home. Behavior modification requires a major time investment by parents and teachers. If they are unwilling to invest the time, behavior modification therapy will be ineffective.

Dr. Hechtman: You mentioned that even though you get a very optimistic drug response on achievement, you don't know how it translates to actual long-term achievements?

Dr. Pelham: I wrote a paper recently (Pelham, 1983) that reviews the literature on the effects of drugs on achievement. There is no long-term, well-controlled study of stimulant drugs, using the low doses now recommended. The Satterfield study does show substantial gains using medication combined with multimodal intervention.

REFERENCES

Abikoff H, Gittelman R: Does behavior therapy normalize the classroom behavior of hyperactive children? Arch Gen Psychiat 1984; 41:449–454.

Atkins M, White K, Pelham WE, Adams P, Case D: Behavioral and pharmacological treatment of a hyperactive, aggressive child. Unpublished manuscript, 1984.

Ayllon T, Laymen D, Kandel HJ: A behavioral-educational alternative to drug control of hyperactive children. J Appl Behav Anal 1975; 8:137–146.

Barkley RA, Cunningham CE: Do stimulant drugs improve the academic performance of hyperkinetic children? Clin Pediatr 1978; 17:85–92.

Birch HG, Demb H: The formation and extinction of conditioned reflexes in "brain-damaged" and mongoloid children. J Nerv Ment Dis 1959: 129:162–170.

Bosco J, Robins S: Hyperkinesis: prevalence and treatment. In C Whalen, B Henker (eds): Hyperactive Children: The Social Ecology of Identification and Treatment. New York, Academic Press, 1980.

Charles L, Schain R: A four-year follow-up study of the effects of methylphenidate on the behavior and academic achievement of hyperactive children. J Abnorm Child Psychol 1981; 9:495–505.

Conners C: A teacher rating scale for use in drug studies with children. Am J Psychiat 1969; 126:884–888.

Gadow KD: Pharmacotherapy for learning disabilities. J Learn Disabil 1983; 16:290–299.

Gittelman R, Abikoff H, Pollack E, Klein DF, Katz S, Mattes J: A controlled trial of behavior modification and methylphenidate in hyperactive children. In CK Whalen, B Henker (eds): Hyperactive Children: The Social Ecology of Identification and Treatment. New York, Academic Press, 1980.

Goyette CH, Conners CK, Ulrich RF: Normative data on revised Conners parent and teacher rating scales. J Abnorm Child Psychol 1978; 6:221–236.

Hinshaw SP, Henker B, Whalen CK: Self-control in hyperactive boys in anger-inducing situations: effects of cognitive-behavioral training and of methylphenidate. J Abnorm Psychol 1985; in press.

Jastak J, Bijou S, Jastak R: Wide Range Achievement Test. Wilmington, DE, Guidance Associates, 1978.

Loney J, Milich R: Development and evaluation of a placebo for studies on operant behavioral intervention. J Behav Ther Exp Psychiat 1978; 9:327–333.

Loney J, Milich R: Pharmacological and behavioral treatment of hyperactivity. Unpublished manuscript, Department of Psychiatry, University of Iowa, 1983.

Mash EJ, McElwee J: Manual for coding interactions. In E Mash, L Terdal (eds): Behavioral Assessment, New York, Springer, 1976.

Mattes JA, Gittelman R: Growth of hyperactive children on maintenance regimen of methylphenidate. Arch Gen Psychiat 1983; 40:317–321.

Milich R, Landau S: Socialization and peer relations in the hyperactive child. In K Gadow, I Bialer (eds): Advances in Learning and Behavioral Disabilities, vol. 1. Greenwich, CT, JAI Press, 1982.

Oden S, Asher S: Coaching children in social skills for friendship making. Child Develop 1977; 48:495–506.

O'Leary SG, Pelham WE: Behavior therapy and withdrawal of stimulant medication with hyperactive children. Pediatrics 1978; 61:211–217.

O'Leary KD, Pelham WE, Rosenbaum A, Price GH: Behavioral treatment of hyperkinetic children: an experimental evaluation of its usefulness. Clin Pediat 1976; 15:510–515.

O'Leary K, Turkewitz H, Ironsmith M: Generalization and maintenance of appropriate behavior through self-control. J Consult Clin Psychol 1975; 43:577–583.

Patterson G: Families: Application of Social Learning to Family Life. Champaign, The Research Press, 1976.

Pelham WE: Withdrawal of a stimulant drug and concurrent behavioral intervention in the treatment of a hyperactive child. Behav Ther 1977; 8:473–479.

Pelham WE: Hyperactive children. In RP Liberman (ed): Symposium on Behavior Therapy in Psychiatry. Psychiatr Clin N Am 1978; 1:227–246.

Pelham WE: Childhood hyperactivity: diagnosis, etiology, nature and treatment. In R Gatchel, A Baum, J Singer (eds): Behavioral Medicine and Clinical Psychology: Overlapping Disciplines. Hillsdale, NJ, Erlbaum, 1982.

Pelham WE: The effects of psychostimulants on academic achievement in hyperactive and learning-disabled children. Thalamus 1983; 3:1–47.

Pelham WE, Bender ME: Peer relationships in hyperactive children: description and treatment. In K Gadow, I Bialer (eds): Advances in Learning and Behavioral Disabilities, vol 1. Greenwich, CT, JAI Press, 1982.

Pelham WE, Bender ME, Caddell JM, Booth S, Moorer S: The dose-response effects of methylphenidate on classroom academic and social behavior in children with attention deficit disorder. Arch Gen Psychiat 1985; 42:948–952.

Pelham WE, Milich R: Peer relations in children with hyperactivity/attention deficit disorder. J Learn Disabil 1984; 17:560–567.

Pelham WE, Murphy HA: Behavioral and pharmacological treatment of attention deficit and conduct disorders. In N Herson (ed.) Pharmacological and Behavioral Treatment: An Integrative Approach, New York, Wiley, 1986.

Pelham W, Schnedler R, Bologna N, Contreras A: Behavioral and stimulant treatment of hyperactive children: A therapy study with methylphenidate probes in a within-subject design. J Appl Behav Anal 1980; 13:221–236.

Riddle D, Rapoport J: A 2-year follow-up of 72 hyperactive boys. J Nerv Ment Dis 1976; 162:126–134.

Satterfield JH, Cantwell DP, Satterfield B: Multimodality treatment: a one-year follow-up of 84 hyperactive boys. Arch Gen Psychiat 1979; 36:965–974.

Satterfield JH, Hoppe CM, Schell AM: A prospective study of delinquency in 110 adolescent boys with attention deficit disorder and 88 normal adolescent boys. Am J Psychiat 1982; 139:795–798.

Sleater E, von Neumann A: Methylphenidate in the treatment of hyperkinetic children. Clin Pediatr 1974; 13:19–24.

Sprague RL, Berger BD: Drug effects on learning performance: Relevance of animal research to pediatric psychopharmacology. In R Knights, D Bakker (eds): Treatment of Hyperactive and Learning Disabled Children. Baltimore, University Park Press, 1980, pp 167–183.

Sprague RL, Sleater EK: Methylphenidate in hyperkinetic children: differences in dose effects on learning and social behavior. Science 1977; 198:1274–1276.

Swanson J, Kinsbourne M: The cognitive effects of stimulant drugs on hyperactive (inattentive) children. In G Hale, M Lewis (eds): Attention and the Development of Cognitive Skills. New York, Plenum, 1979.

Weiss G, Kruger E, Danielson U, Elman M: Effects of long-term treatment of hyperactive children with methylphenidate. Can Med Assoc J 1975; 112:159–165.

Werry J, Sprague R, Cohen M: Conners Teacher Rating Scale for use in drug studies with children—an empirical study. J Abnorm Child Psychol 1975; 3:217–229.

4

Brain Event-related Potentials in Evaluation of Cognitive Deficits in Attention Deficit Disorder and Outcome of Stimulant Therapy

RAFAEL KLORMAN, LEONARD F. SALZMAN AND
AGNETA D. BORGSTEDT

In 1977, we began a research program employing brain event-related potentials (ERP) to assess cognitive deficits in children with attention deficit disorder (ADD) and the treatment of these disturbances by stimulant medication. At that time, a consensus was emerging—which has since been codified in DSM-III—that cognitive disorder is a central feature of this syndrome. Indeed, several overviews of the voluminous literature have documented the prevalence of attentional disturbances and impulsivity in ADD children (e.g., Rosenthal and Allen, 1978; Sroufe, 1975). In addition recent reviews make it clear that the reduction of these cognitive deficits is among the most salient improvements brought about by stimulant therapy of ADD patients (Aman, 1978; Conners and Werry, 1979; Rosenthal and Allen, 1978; Sroufe, 1975).

THE CONTINUOUS PERFORMANCE TEST

Although many methodologies have been employed in the study of cognitive disorder in ADD, one of the most commonly used techniques in this research has been the Continuous Performance Test (CPT), originally developed by Rosvold and his colleagues (Rosvold *et al.*, 1956). Figure 4.1 depicts the three versions of this test used in our work. In all versions, the subject views a display of briefly presented characters that appear singly, in unpredictable order, and at brief intervals (usually 1-2 seconds). In one form of the test, one character—usually the letter X—is designated as the target, or a rare event, occurring on 10% to 15% of all trials and to which

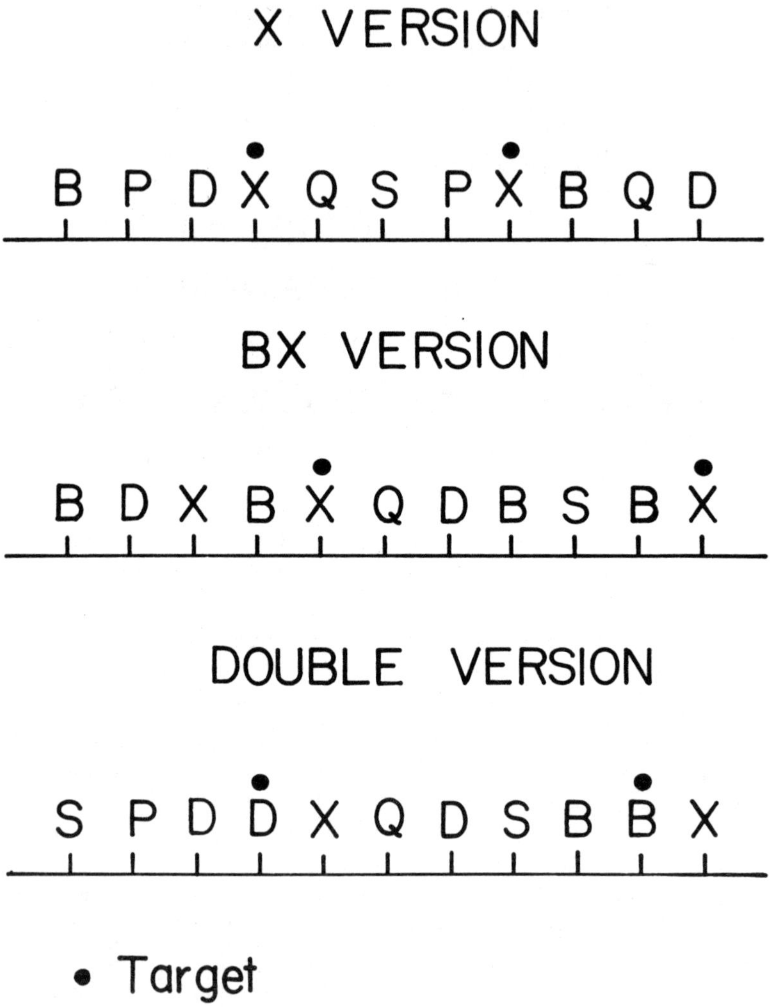

FIG. 4.1 Diagrammatic representation of three versions of the Continuous Performance Test. Each vertical line depicts the presentation of the letter displayed above it. Depending on the study, stimuli are displayed for periods of 50 to 200 msec and at intervals ranging between 1 to 2 secs. For each format of the task, the filled circles designate the target searched for by the subject.

a button press is required. This format of the test is depicted in Figure 4.1, where it is designated the X version.

In a second and more difficult form of the test, the target is defined as only those occurrences of X that are preceded by another letter, e.g., B. The BX version of CPT places a greater memory load on the subject than

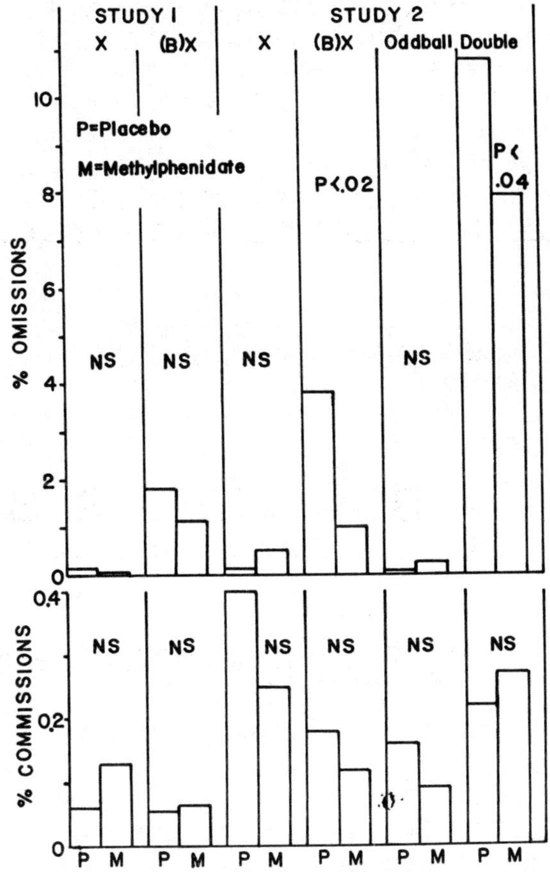

FIG. 4.2 Percentage of omissions and commissions in various tasks presented to normal young adults challenged with placebo (P) and methylphenidate (M). A floor effect operated for most tasks and only for the two most difficult tests, CPT-BX and CPT-Double in Study 2, did methylphenidate reduce omission errors. All other differences are nonsignificant. (Reproduced from Coons *et al.* [1981] with permission of Elsevier Scientific Publishers, Ireland.)

does the X version, in that correct performance requires discriminating among occurrences of X, depending on the preceding stimulus.

An even more difficult version of this test was developed by Friedman and his associates (Friedman *et al.*, 1978). In this format of CPT, which we have dubbed CPT Double, the subject is required to press a button whenever any letter is repeated. The cognitive load is increased, relative to CPT-BX, because the subject needs to consider any letter, not only X, as a potential target.

At this point, the reader unfamiliar with this literature may wonder why so many versions of CPT are necessary. The reason is that these tasks generate different rates of errors. For instance, in a recent study from our laboratory (Coons *et al.*, 1981), college students tested under placebo missed 0.1% of targets in CPT-X, 3.8% under CPT-BX, and 10.8% under CPT-Double (cf. Figure 4.2). Of course, the error rate, i.e., the difficulty of the test, is affected by the characteristics of the population studied (e.g., age and clinical status) as well as various conditions of administration (e.g., frequency of targets and task duration). (Davies and Parasuraman (1981) provide a comprehensive review of the effect of these factors on error rates in vigilance tests.) Thus, there have been occasional reports of failures to detect differences on this test among subsets of ADD compared with normal children, or subjects tested under stimulants compared with placebo (Coons *et al.*, 1981; Michael *et al.*, 1981; O'Dougherty *et al.*, 1984; Sostek *et al.*, 1980).

From a psychometric standpoint, one might observe that even if CPT taps fundamental cognitive deficits of ADD children and the enhancing effects of stimulants, these effects could be obscured by a too easy version of the task. This is an issue to which we will return later. For now we wish to emphasize the importance of utilizing tests that are sufficiently challenging for the target population.

BRAIN EVENT RELATED POTENTIALS (ERPS)

Over the past two decades, a plethora of studies has documented the sensitivity of ERPs to attentional processes. This work, summarized in a number of recent reviews (e.g., Donchin and McCarthy, 1979; Picton and Stuss, 1980; Pritchard, 1981), has supported the view that ERP components are sensitive manifestations of cognitive events.

At the time that we began our research on ADD, it seemed intuitively promising to examine ADD children's ERPs during cognitive processing, insofar as cognitive deficits were viewed as the hallmark of the disorder. A second appeal of this strategy was the similarity of CPT to paradigms utilized in ERP research. Hence, we decided to investigate ERP during CPT-X in unmedicated normal children as well as ADD patients challenged with placebo and methylphenidate.

CLINICAL CHALLENGE STUDY 1

Samples

Our initial investigation (Klorman *et al.*, 1979) employed 18 ADD boys from the practice of a pediatric neurologist (ADB). For this and subsequent clinical studies, all patients were diagnosed by procedures including: extended neurologic examinations (Paine and Oppe, 1966; Kinsbourne, 1973); waking clinical EEGs; laboratory tests; and consultations

TABLE 4.1 *Characteristics of ADD and normal children in Clinical Challenge Study 1*

	Age[a]		Home activity scale[b,c]	
	Mean	± SD	Mean	± SD
ADD ($N = 18$)	9.53	1.38	1.24	0.78
Normal ($N = 17$)	9.60	1.20	0.27	0.14

Note. Adapted from Klorman *et al.* (1979) with permission of the Society for Psychophysiological Research.

Statistical tests compare ADD and normal children.

[a] Not significant.

[b] $p < 0.001$.

[c] Scored 0–4.

with teachers and parents to review the child's current functioning and pediatric history. These diagnostic procedures were intended to rule out other medical, neurologic, or psychiatric conditions that might account for the observed disturbances. In our initial study, the ADD cohort consisted of children with a history of positive response to methylphenidate therapy. Patients were tested in the summer after discontinuing medication for at least 2 weeks. Their parents were interviewed by a clinical psychologist (RK) concerning the items of the Home Activity Scale (Werry and Sprague, 1970) during the washout period. In addition, they completed the Conners (1976) Parent Questionnaire.

A comparison sample of 17 normal children was drawn from the university community. As shown in Table 4.1, normal and ADD children were comparable in age but, as expected, parents described the clinical sample as sigificantly more hyperactive and distractible than their normal peers.

Procedures

In this study ADD patients were tested twice. On one occasion, they received a capsule containing lactose and, on the other, methylphenidate (0.3 mg/kg). In this, as in all of our investigations, capsules were administered in a double-blind format, random order, and following at least 2 hours of fasting. Testing did not begin for 90 minutes after the capsules were ingested. In subsequent studies, we have imposed a similar delay between the ingestion of the assigned capsule and the beginning of testing. This interval was taken up by the attachment of electrodes and informal interactions between subject and experimenter. The duration of this period was calculated so as to promote the significant absorption of methylphenidate (Perel and Dayton, 1978) as well as familiarization with the laboratory setting.

Normal children participated in a single session, identical in all details to the testing of ADD patients, except for the omission of any capsules.

All comparisons with the normal sample involved the ADD children's placebo testing.

Although other procedures were administered, the most interesting results emerged from the X version of CPT, which was administered for 5 minutes and with 1-second intervals between presentations of letters. The instructions emphasized speed as well as accuracy. As in all our subsequent research, the children received brief practice in the task before the test began.

Results: Performance

As shown in Figure 4.3, ADD patients when tested under placebo, missed nearly four times as many targets as did normal children (omission errors, $p < 0.001$). Similarly, they made approximately four times more inappropriate button presses to nontargets than did the normal boys (commission errors, $p < 0.001$). Finally, the reaction times of ADD

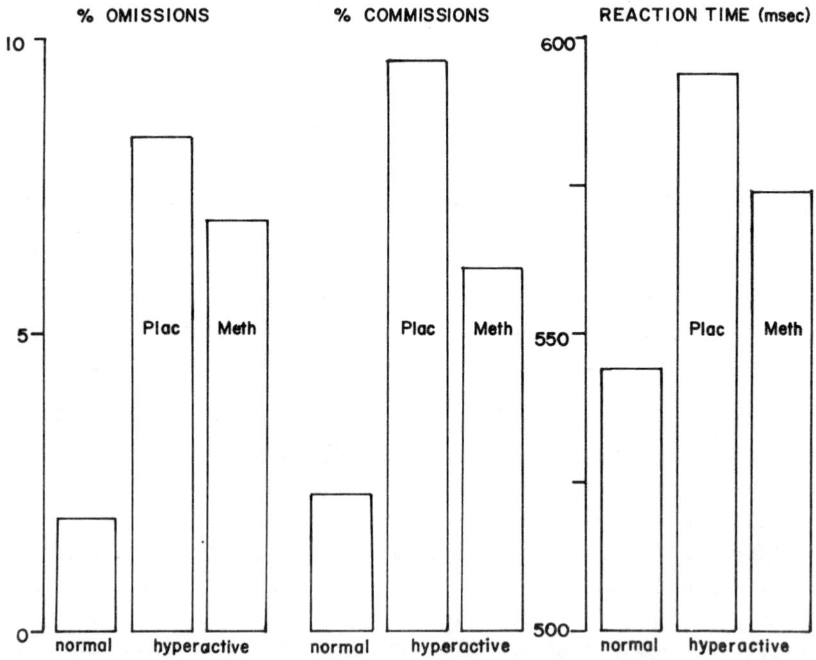

FIG. 4.3 Results for performance measures in Clinical Challenge Study 1 for normal and ADD (hyperactive) samples. Placebo (Plac) treated ADD children displayed higher rates of omission and commission errors as well as slower reaction times than normal children. Methylphenidate (Meth) significantly reduced commission errors and reaction time. (Adapted from Klorman *et al.* [1979] with permission of the Society for Psychophysiological Research.)

patients were significantly slower than their normal counterparts ($p < 0.02$).

As is also shown in Figure 4.3, the single dose of methylphenidate reduced all of these deficits, the improvements being significant for commission errors ($p < 0.04$) and reaction time ($p < 0.05$). Thus, there was evidence that the stimulant normalized the ADD child's performance on CPT, an observation reported many times before (e.g., Aman, 1978).

Results: ERP

Figure 4.4 displays some individual examples of the average vertex EEG response to targets and nontargets. These responses contained a positive wave that peaked around 250 to 500 msec after the letters were presented. We identified this peak as the late positive component (LPC) previously described in the literature as reflecting evaluation aspects of cognitive processing. Indeed, as illustrated in Figure 4.4, for both normal and ADD children, this wave achieved larger amplitude following the experimentally more salient stimuli, i.e., targets ($p < 0.03$). Notably, placebo-treated ADD children displayed smaller-amplitude LPC than did their normal counterparts ($p < 0.03$). Moreover, methylphenidate significantly increased the ADD sample's LPC amplitude ($p < 0.05$). Thus, the results for this important ERP wave paralleled those for performance, i.e., normalization of the ADD patient's responses by methylphenidate.

Although these findings were provocative, they required replication and extension. A review of the literature on ERP research in ADD had emphasized the many instances of failure to replicate results in this area (Shagass *et al.*, 1978). In addition, the results were based on a sample of drug-responsive patients. It seemed appropriate to inquire whether ADD patients, not previously medicated, would display similar responses. These questions were examined in our second study.

CLINICAL CHALLENGE STUDY 2

Samples

This study (Michael *et al.*, 1981) included a sample of 29 ADD children, 17 of whom, like our previous clinical sample, were withdrawn from stimulant therapy before participating in the research. The remainder were newly referred patients who had never before received a stimulant. As in Study 1, all patients were drawn from Dr. Borgstedt's private practice and subjected to extensive evaluations to eliminate alternative diagnoses. All patients scored above 1.05 on the Home Activity Scale (0 = not at all, 4 = extremely), whereas new referrals also exceeded Sprague's (Sprague *et al.*, 1974; Sprague, personal communication) recommended cutoffs for the

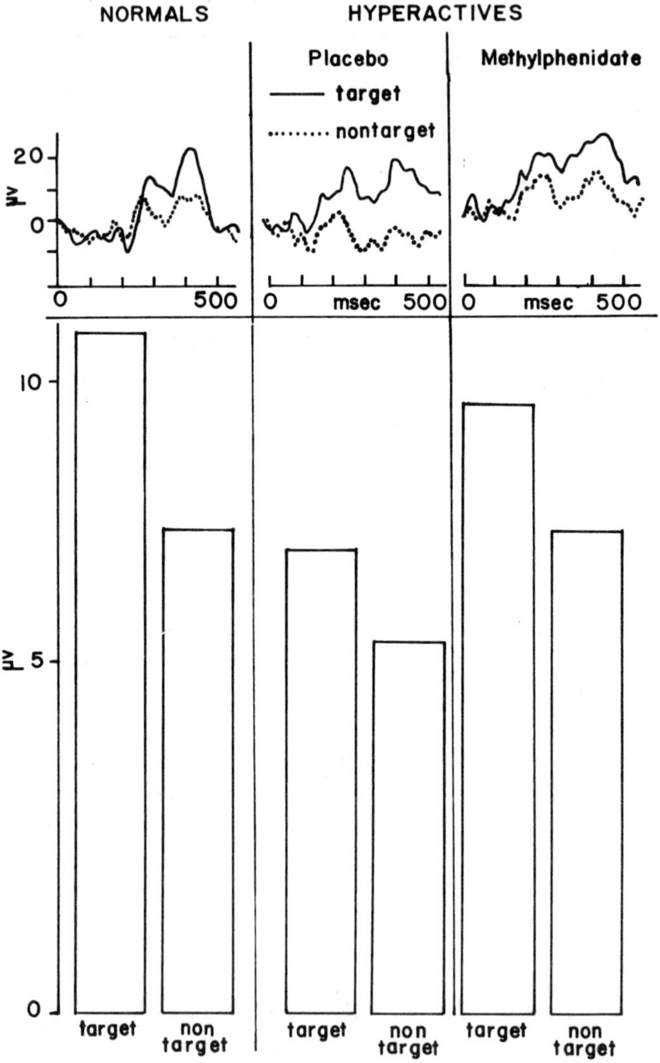

FIG. 4.4 Results for Event Related Potentials (ERP) in Clinical Challenge Study 1. The top panel depicts individual examples of ERPs to targets (solid line) and nontargets (dashed line) for one normal subject and an ADD (hyperactive) patient tested under placebo and methylphenidate. Positivity at the vertex electrode is displayed upward. The late positive component (LPC) was identified as the most positive wave in the interval 250 to 500 msec post-stimulus onset. The lower bar graph depicts mean LPC amplitude for each sample and pharacologic condition. Targets evoked larger LPC amplitude than nontargets. Normals displayed larger amplitude than ADD patients tested under placebo. Methylphenidate augmented ADD patients' LPC amplitude. (Adapted from Klorman *et al.* [1979] with permission of the Society for Psychophysiological Research.)

TABLE 4.2 *Characteristics of ADD and normal children in Clinical Challenge Study 2*

Measure		ADD Patients All	ADD Patients Matched	Normals
Male/Females[a]		25/4	18/3	18/3
Acute/chronic		12/17	10/11	—
Placebo first/second		16/13	10/11	—
Age[a]	$\bar{X}$	9.11	9.31	9.35
	SD	1.96	1.92	1.94
Home activity scale[b]	$\bar{X}$	1.80	1.77	0.49
	SD	0.59	0.44	0.17
Abbreviated Conners	$\bar{X}$	1.87	1.89	0.40
Teacher Scale[b,c]	SD	0.41	0.44	0.41

[a] Nonsignificant difference between ADD and normal children.
[b] Significant ($p < 0.001$) difference between ADD and normal children.
[c] This comparison is based on acute patients and their normal matches.
Note. Reproduced from Michael *et al.* (1981) with permission of the Society for Psychophysiological Research.

Conners (1976) Abbreviated Teacher Scale. (Following Sprague, these cutoffs were 2.3 for third grade ADD-H patients and 1.5 for all other patients. The corresponding cutoff scales used for the normal scale were 1.5 and 1.0, respectively. These values placed normal subjects within 1 *SD* of the mean for other normal samples.) Both sets of cutoffs represented 2 *SD* above normal children's means.

A sample of 21 normal children was obtained, each of whom obtained scores below preset cutoffs on the Home Activity Scale and the teacher's ratings on the Conners Abbreviated Teacher Scale. A subset of the ADD cohort was matched to normal children with regard to gender and age. The samples' characteristics are displayed in Table 4.2. As in Study 1, ADD patients were judged significantly more disturbed than their normal peers.

Procedures

All children were tested on two occasions. ADD patients received 0.3 mg/kg methylphenidate in one session and placebo in the other. Drug administration was multiple-blind and randomly ordered. Normal children did not receive capsules. Contrasts between clinical and normal samples involved placebo data for each ADD child and the comparable session—first or second—for his/her normal match.

All sessions were identical, except for pharmacologic procedures. For all children, fasting was required for two hours before the experiment and there ensued a 90-minute interval before the testing began. The main procedural differences from the preceding study were that CPT-X was administered in two, rather than one, 5-minute phases and was followed by two phases of CPT-BX. To simplify the presentation, results for the two phases combined are reported. A further departure from the earlier work was that instructions emphasized accuracy over speed. (Subsequent studies also employed an accuracy, rather than a speed, set. A further difference from the first study was the inclusion of a midparietal as well as a vertex EEG lead. In more recent work we have also included a midfrontal placement.)

Performance: Differences Between Samples

The results for performance were very similar to those of the previous study. As indicated in Figures 4.5 and 4.6, for the two tasks ADD children missed more targets ($p < 0.003$) and made more commission errors ($p < 0.004$) than did normal children.

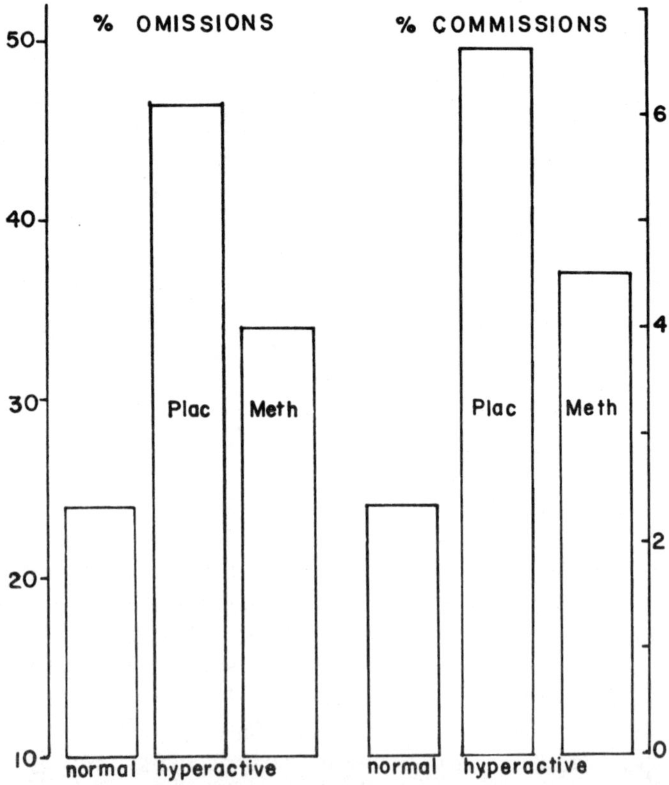

FIG. 4.5 Omission and commission errors in CPT-X, for normal and ADD (hyperactive) children in Clinical Challenge Study 2. Normal children made fewer errors of both types than did ADD patients and methylphenidate decreased both aspects of ADD children's performance. (Adapted from Michael *et al.* [1981] with permission of the Society for Psychophysiological Research.)

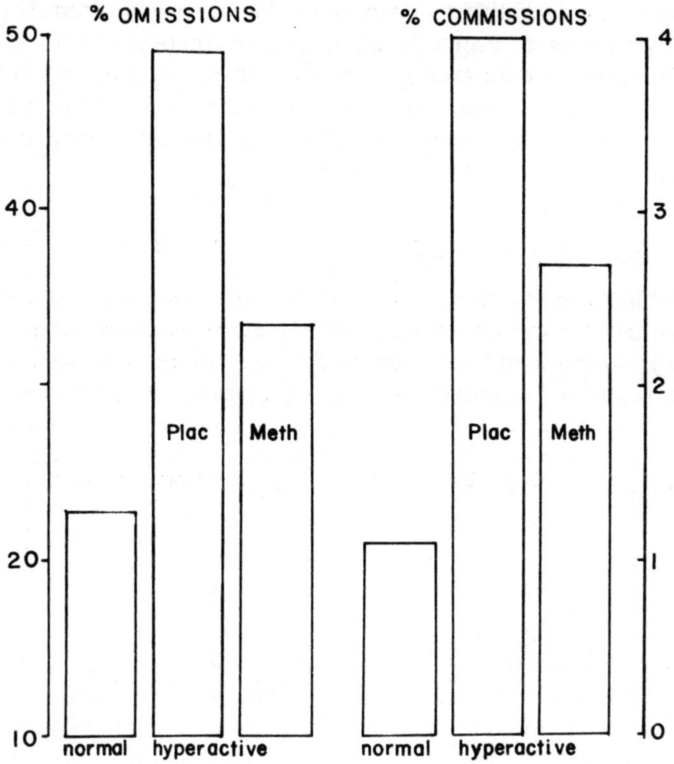

FIG. 4.6 Omission and commission errors in CPT-BX for normals and ADD (hyperactive) children in Clinical Challenge Study 2. The results were similar to those for CPT-X, as described in the text and Figure 4.5. (Adapted from Michael *et al.* [1981] with permission of the Society for Psychophysiological Research.)

At least two other features of the figures deserve mention. First, both groups of children made more errors on the BX version of the test ($p < 0.003$ for omissions and $p < 0.03$ for commissions). Nevertheless, ADD patients performed worse than normals on both tasks. Second, the error rate was considerably higher than in the preceding study. This result was due in part to the inclusion of a much wider age range in this sample (5.9-13.0 vs. 7.0-11.9). Because younger children made more errors of omission ($p < 0.001$) as well as commission ($p < 0.008$), the average rates of errors were quite high. However, when the sample was divided into three levels of age (5.9-8.2, 8.3,-10.4, and 10.6-13.0), normal children at each age level outperformed their ADD counterparts. For instance, omission rates on CPT-BX for placebo-treated ADD and normal children, listed in ascending levels of age, were 62.3% vs. 32.3%, 56.2% vs. 16.0%, and 28.0% vs. 16.3%, respectively.

Further, it is unwarranted to conclude that the youngest ADD children were performing at a chance level. Because targets are relatively infrequent, the ADD group's average omission rate of 49.1% on CPT-BX is the equivalent of 5.7% of all stimuli. Their mean error rate for nontargets, i.e., commission errors, was only 3.5%. Their error rate was 9.2% misclassifications of all stimuli in the session.

Admittedly, though, the error rates for this ADD sample were higher than those reported in other investigations employing CPT (e.g., Sykes *et al.*, 1971; Rapoport *et al.*, 1980). Besides our inclusion of younger subjects in the sample, several characteristics of our versions of CPT increased the task's difficulty. These factors include our use of short intertrial intervals (1 vs. the usual 2 seconds), longer tasks (two blocks of 5 minutes vs. the more common 2 or 3 minutes), and a long overall session. As discussed in the section on the Continuous Performance Test, our choice of moderately difficult tests was based on the concern that easy versions may prove insensitive for older or more skillful subjects.

Performance: Pharmacologic Effects

As illustrated in Figures 4.5 and 4.6, methylphenidate reduced the rate of omission ($p < 0.001$), as well as commission errors ($p < 0.02$). This improvement in accuracy was even more pronounced after eliminating the oldest patients for whom the tests were considerably less difficult. Therefore, all data plotted in Figures 4.5 to 4.8 are based on subjects under 11 years of age. (As detailed in the original report, there was a trend for subjects to benefit from practice independently of the drug administration [$p < 0.05$.] After excluding the oldest group of children, for whom the tasks were least challenging, the magnitude of this effect was considerably diminished).

ERP Results

Figures 4.7 and 4.8 show that the amplitude of the late positive component (LPC) of both ADD and normal children's ERP was systematically related to stimulus relevance. Thus, among both samples and in both tasks, larger LPC amplitude was evoked by target stimuli. As previously found, ADD children displayed smaller LPC amplitude than their normal peers in both tasks, this diagnostic difference being more pronounced when older children were excluded.

The pharmacologic results for CPT-X replicated those in Study 1. As shown in Figure 4.7 methylphenidate increased LPC amplitude to task stimuli, an effect that was greater among younger subjects ($p < 0.005$). However, we did not find a comparable enhancement of LPC in CPT-BX,

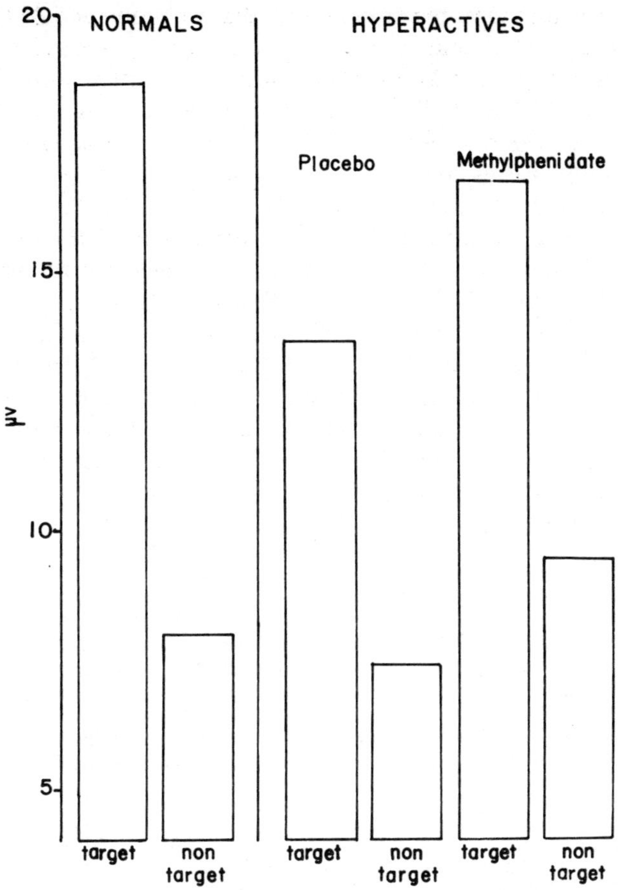

FIG. 4.7 Mean LPC amplitude at the vertex in CPT-X for normal and hyperactive (ADD) samples in Clinical Challenge Study 2. The results were very similar to those in Clinical Challenge Study 1, as described in the text and Figure 4.4. (Adapted from Michael *et al.* [1981] with permission of the Society for Psychophysiological Research.)

perhaps because of an unexpected effect of drug order and a fortuitous reduction of thc sample size as a result of equipment problems.

Discussion

The main contribution of Study 2 was the replication of Study 1 in a larger and more representative clinical sample. Separate analyses disclosed that newly referred, as well as previously medicated patients, responded similarly to the pharmacologic challenge. Specifically, methylphenidate increased their accuracy and enhanced the amplitude of their LPC in tasks requiring sustained attention.

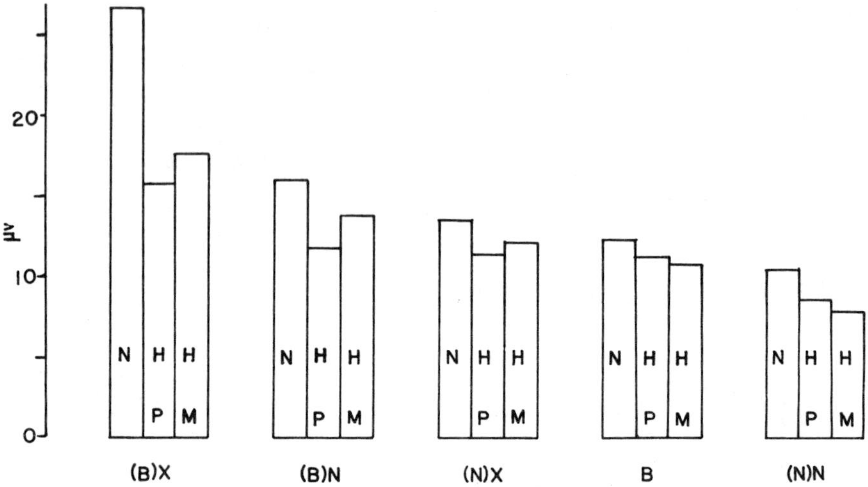

FIG. 4.8 Mean LPC amplitude at the vertex in CPT-BX for normal (N) and ADD (H) samples in Clinical Challenge Study 2. Pharmacologic conditions are coded P for placebo and M for methylphenidate. Target stimuli, the letter X preceded by B, (B)X, evoked the largest LPC amplitude for both samples. Nontargets were divided into four categories: (1) any letter other than X preceded by B, (B)N; (2) any occurrence of X not preceded by B, (N)X; (3) all presentations of B, B; and (4) any letter other than X that was not preceded by B, (N)N. Normals exhibited larger LPC to targets than placebo-treated ADD patients. The slight increase in LPC amplitude to targets under methylphenidate was not significant. (Adapted from Michael *et al.* [1981] with permission of the Society for Psychophysiological Research.)

As was the case in Study 1, even after the enhancing effects of stimulant medication there remained differences between normals and ADD children. Thus, we have followed Halliday's (Halliday *et al.*, 1976) terminology of "normalization" to refer to these positive effects.

A second finding consistent with the initial study is that diagnostic and pharmacologic differences in LPC amplitude involved both targets as well as nontargets. At first blush, these results would appear to suggest a nonspecific effect of arousal and to rule out selective attention. Closer analysis, however, militates against such a conclusion. First, ERP studies involving passive visual stimulation procedures not requiring procedures not requiring attention have not yielded uniform differences between ADD and normal samples or stimulant and placebo trials (cf., review by Shagass *et al.*, 1978). Our own work with passive presentations of the same stimuli employed in CPT yielded very small LPC amplitude, which did not vary between clinical samples or pharmacologic states (Klorman *et al.*, 1979; Michael *et al.*, 1981).

Further insight into this matter comes from recognizing that applying the term nontarget in the present task is arbitrary and somewhat misleading. CPT differs considerably from selective attention paradigms in which the relevant and irrelevant stimuli differ in sensory modality (e.g., auditory vs. visual), input channel (e.g., right vs. left ear), or physical intensity (e.g., loud vs. soft tones). In order to perform correctly on CPT, a subject must allocate considerable capacity to identifying nontargets as well as targets. Hence, nontargets should not be viewed as irrelevant or involving automatic processes. Thus, it makes theoretical sense that there are diagnostic and pharmacologic differences in ERP components that reflect capacity allocation to nontargets.

We have already commented extensively on the moderating effect of task difficulty and age on these results. We have proposed that a sufficient level of psychological challenge must be presented for the detection of diagnostic differences or stimulant effects (Coons *et al.*, 1981). A similar point was made in Weiss and Laties' (1962) now classic review of the effects of amphetamines on adults. They noted that stimulants yielded enhanced performance in vigilance tasks of sufficiently long duration to evoke degradation of performance under placebo. The importance of the difficulty level of a task as well as other factors in the detection of psychological deficits is also highlighted in Chapman and Chapman's (1973) careful analysis of this topic.

STUDIES WITH NORMAL YOUNG ADULTS

The importance of a task's level of difficulty in the detection of stimulant effects was underscored by the results of our work with normal young adults. We studied three samples of young adults screened for medical and psychiatric conditions not indicating for the administration of stimulants (Coons *et al.*, 1981; Klorman *et al.*, 1984; Strauss *et al.*, 1984).

Procedures and Results

Subjects were tested under conditions nearly identical to those of ADD children in our Clinical Challenge Study 2. These included fasting conditions before each capsule; double-blind, randomly ordered drug administration; an active dose of 0.3 mg/kg; and a 75 to 90 minute interval between capsule ingestion and the onset of testing. The results for performance in the first two studies are shown in Figure 4.2. In the first study we failed to find any effect of this stimulant on performance in CPT-X or CPT-BX. Analogously, there were no pharmacologic effects on the concomitant LPC in these tasks, although target stimuli evoked the predicted trend of larger LPC amplitude to targets than nontargets ($p < 0.001$). Reasoning that these tasks were too easy for these adult subjects the experiment was repeated and the more difficult double version

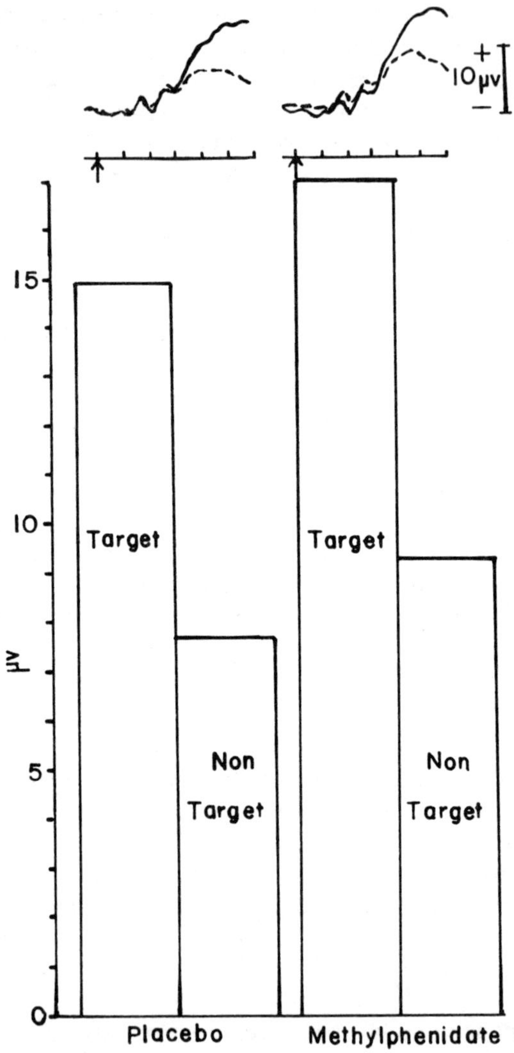

FIG. 4.9 The top panel depicts the grand mean ERP at the mid parietal lead to targets (solid line) and nontargets (dashed line) in CPT double for normal young adults challenged with placebo and methylphenidate. The arrow denotes stimulus onset and the abscissa is demarcated in 100-msec intervals. Methylphenidate resulted in significant increases in the amplitude of LPC evoked by targets and nontargets. (Reproduced from Coons *et al.* [1981] with permission of Elsevier Scientific Publishers, Ireland.)

of CPT was added. In Study 2, once again, nearly error-free performance was obtained in CPT-X and there were no stimulant effects on accuracy or LPC. CPT-BX was administered in a longer format (8 vs. 5 minutes) than in the initial study, a factor which increased the error rate and perhaps accounted for the observed reduction in omission errors under methylphenidate ($p < 0.02$), cf. Figure 4.2). However, LPC amplitude in CPT-BX was unaffected by the stimulant.

In contrast to the preceding results, CPT-double evoked a much higher rate of errors, nearly 10%. As predicted for this more challenging task, the stimulant resulted in a significant reduction of omission errors ($p < 0.04$) as well as augmentation of LPC amplitude ($p < 0.02$). These effects on LPC are illustrated in Figure 4.9.

Discussion

In combination, these results suggested that a moderate level of task difficulty, or capacity allocation, is required for the detection of enhancing effects by methylphenidate. Of course, if a task is too easy, a floor effect operates on errors and it is not possible to demonstrate increases in accuracy. However, floor effects did not operate for LPC or reaction time in the less challenging versions of CPT. In fact, even for CPT-double, reaction time was improved only marginally by methylphenidate.

This reasoning implied that raising the difficulty level of CPT-double should further increase the advantage of the stimulant over placebo. Therefore in our third challenge study, the difficulty of CPT-double was increased by lengthening its duration from two blocks of 5 minutes to an uninterrupted vigil of 45 minutes. As shown in Figure 4.10, when subjects received this protracted test under placebo, they became increasingly less accurate and slower ($p < 0.0001$). As expected, this impairment of performance over the vigil was greatly reduced by the stimulant challenge ($p < 0.03$). Further, as shown in Figure 4.11, LPC amplitude tended to decrease or remain stable over the course of the placebo vigil, whereas it increased under methylphenidate ($p < 0.0008$). Finally, the latency of this peak, currently held to represent evaluation time, was slower under placebo, especially as the vigil wore on. In combination, these findings suggest that methylphenidate retarded the deterioration of performance in a challenging vigilance task by reducing the concomitant increases in stimulus evaluation time over the course of the vigil ($p < 0.007$).

Additional implications from this work relate to the generality of the stimulant's enhancing effects across development. For a long time, the belief has prevailed that these positive effects are limited to ADD children, presumably because of aberrant levels of arousal or a developmental lag. However, as noted by Sroufe (1975), the view that ADD children have a paradoxic reaction to stimulants is contradicted by firm and extensive evidence that adults profit in similar ways from these substances (Weiss and Laties, 1962; Rapoport *et al.*, 1980). The three studies summarized above provide further support for the similarity of stimulant effects on the sustained attention of adults and children. More recently, Rapoport *et al.*

(1980) provided further evidence of the generality of these effects by showing their existence in normal as well as ADD children and in normal young adults.

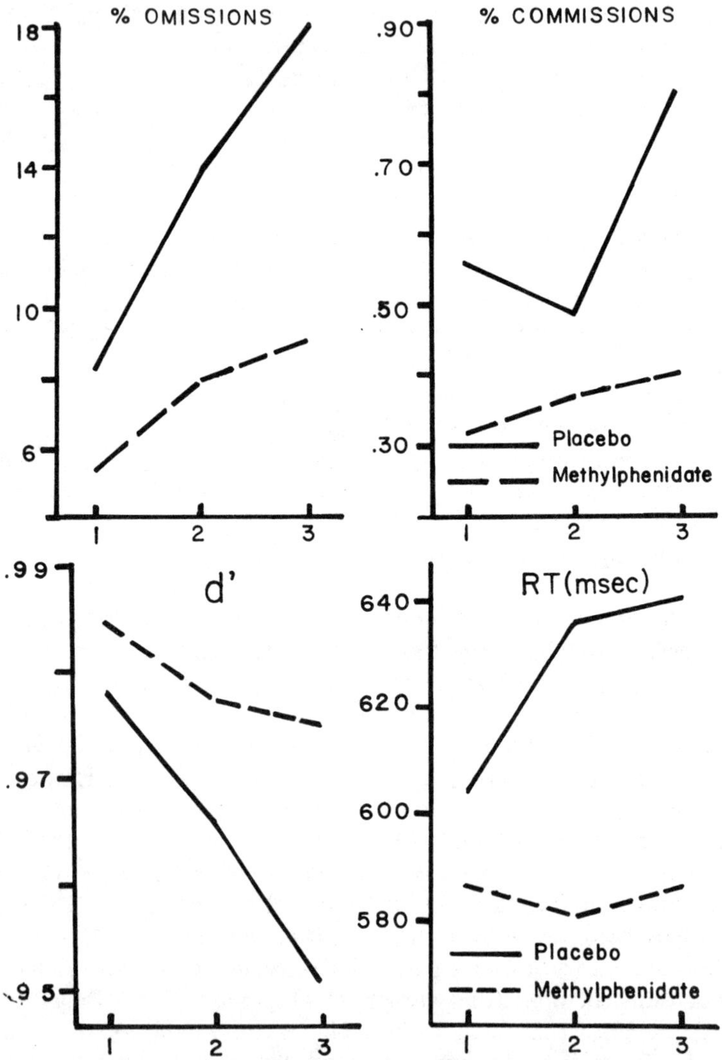

FIG. 4.10 Performance measures in our third challenge study with normal adults. Data are displayed as means for consecutive 15-min intervals in the vigil (CPT-Double). Percent omission errors percent commission errors, sensitivity of detection (d′) and reaction time in msec deteriorated over the placebo vigil. Methylphenidate attenuated this impairment in performance. Note that d′ was computed by Grier's (1971) distribution-free formulas and can range from a minimum of 0 to a maximum of 1. (Reproduced from Strauss *et al.* [1985] with permission of the Society for Psychophysiology Research.)

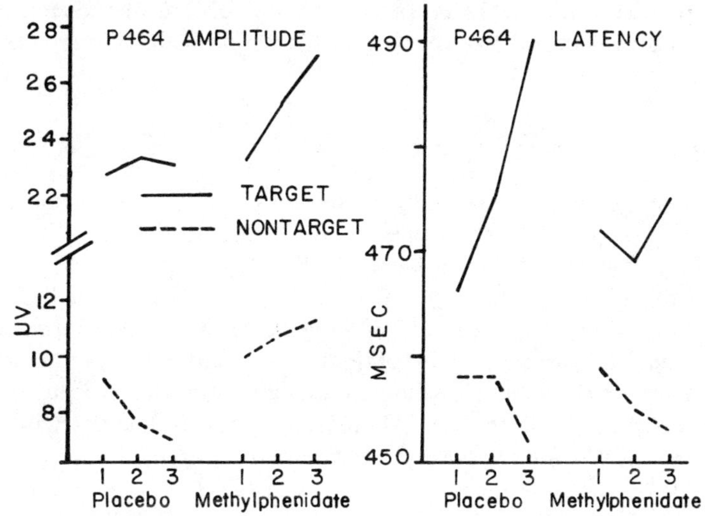

FIG. 4.11 Mean amplitude and latency of the parietal P464 component over consecutive thirds of the vigil. Methylphenidate reduced the amplitude diminution and latency slowing of P464 that took place over the course of the placebo vigil. (Reproduced from Strauss *et al.* [1984] with permission of the Society for Psychophysiological Research.)

DUAL DOSE CLINICAL CHALLENGE STUDY 3

Introduction

At the same time as the above studies with adults were conducted, we performed a third clinical challenge study (Klorman *et al.*, 1983). Several questions were examined. First, in our previous work we had employed a single dose of methylphenidate, 0.3 mg/kg. This choice was based on reports (Werry and Sprague, 1974; Sprague and Sleator, 1975, 1977) that the behavior of ADD children improved monotonically with dose levels over the range of 0.1 to 1 mg/kg, whereas cognitive performance was optimized by medium dose levels, e.g., 0.3 mg/kg. Therefore, we sought to compare the differential effects of two dose levels—the theoretically optimal dose used in our previous work as well as the highest dose likely to be tolerated without unpleasant side effects (0.6 mg/kg).

A second question concerned the generality of the previously observed effects across levels of clinical disturbance. Therefore, we examined a sample of patients who fell short of our research criteria for ADD but for whom stimulant therapy was prescribed.

The third question stemmed from a growing consensus in the field that LPC is not a unitary process but is composed of multiple waves (Picton and Stuss, 1980; Friedman *et al.*, 1981; Sutton and Ruchkin, 1981). Our previous work with ADD children had not differentiated among these waves, and we attempted to determine which LPC components were affected by stimulants.

Samples

Forty-one patients were referred to the research by a pediatric neurologist, Dr. Agneta Borstedt, and a child psychiatrist, Dr. Werner Halpern. Twenty-seven of these patients met the criteria for ADD at home and school, detailed in the section on samples in Clinical Challenge Study 2. Another 14 fell short of meeting one or both of these criteria. As noted above, these borderline ADD patients were judged as sufficiently disturbed by their physicians to warrant a trial of stimulants. Fourteen of the former, or cross-situational, ADD patients were matched pairwise with the borderline ADDs for purposes of comparisons. Table 4.3 describes these two samples.

Procedures

In this study, patients participated in three sessions at the beginning of one of which they received placebo, 0.3 mg/kg methylphenidate, or 0.6 mg/kg. Subjects were randomly assigned to one of the six possible drug orders. Otherwise, all pharmacologic procedures were the same as in the preceding challenge studies.

TABLE 4.3 *Characteristics of cross-situational and borderline ADD patients in Clinical Challenge Study 3*

Measure		Cross-situational ADD		
		All	Matched	Borderline
Male/female[a]		19/8	12/2	12/2
Placebo session: 1st/2nd/3rd[a]		8/11/8	5/5/4	6/4/4
Age (yr)[a]	$\bar{X}$	8.34	8.78	9.00
	SD	1.28	1.12	1.08
WISC IQ[a]	$\bar{X}$	105.00	104.92	104.08
	SD	12.11	10.46	11.89
Home Activity	$\bar{X}$	1.96	1.70	1.25
Scale*	SD	0.56	0.48	0.63
Abbreviated Teacher Conners	$\bar{X}$	1.98	1.95	1.51
Scale*	SD	0.41	0.48	0.54

[a] Not significant.
* $p < 0.05$.
Note. Reproduced from Klorman *et al.* (1983) with permission of Elsevier Scientific Publishers, Ireland.
All comparisons are between matched ADD and borderline patients.

The main experimental tasks were the X and double versions of CPT, which were administered, respectively, in one and two 6.25-minutes trial blocks. Practice in each task was conducted before testing began and instructions emphasized accuracy over speed.

Results: *Performance*

Figure 4.12 displays the results for cross-situational patients' performance in this task. In both tasks, methylphenidate reduced the rate of omissions ($p < 0.0001$) and commissions ($p < 0.007$). Medication also improved reaction time ($p < 0.0003$). It is evident, though, that for cross-situational subjects stimulant medication increased speed only in the easier task. Interestingly, there were no significant differences in the improvement of performance brought about by the two doses, a finding consistent with Sprague and Sleator's reports (1975, 1977). Finally, matched cross-situational and borderline patients' peformance benefited to a similar extent from methylphenidate.

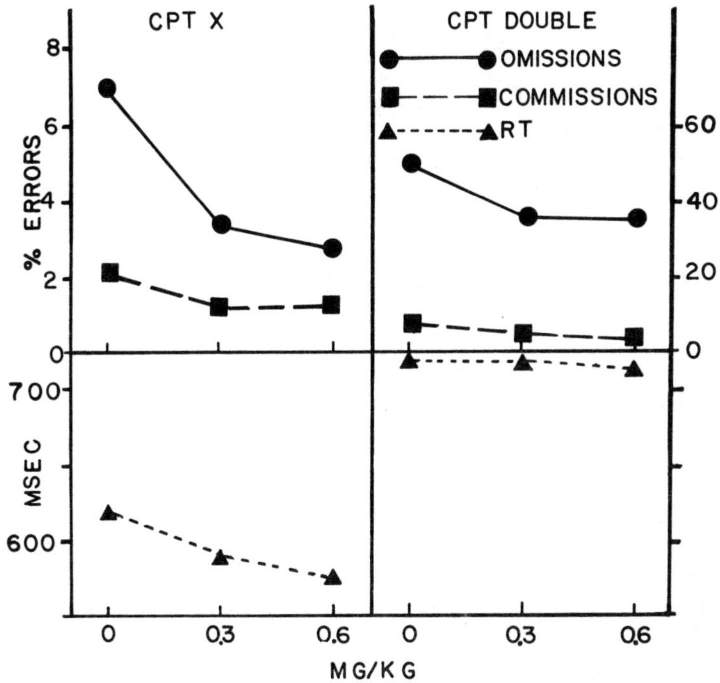

FIG. 4.12 Percentage errors and mean reaction time for cross-situational ADD patients in Clinical Challenge Study 3. For both CPT-X and CPT-Double challenges of 0.3 and 0.6 mg/kg methylphenidate resulted in comparable, reduction of errors and speed. (Reproduced from Klorman *et al.* [1983] with permission of Elsevier Scientific Publishers, Ireland.

The comments under the Samples section of Clinical Challenge Study 2 concerning error rates in CPT apply also to these results. It is evident that the double version of CPT resulted in a high rate of missed targets under placebo. Significant drug-induced increases in accuracy were obtained in both the easy and difficult versions of CPT. Examination of individual records, however, reveals that, for many children, one task was too difficult or the other too easy. Clearly, unless a large sample is used,

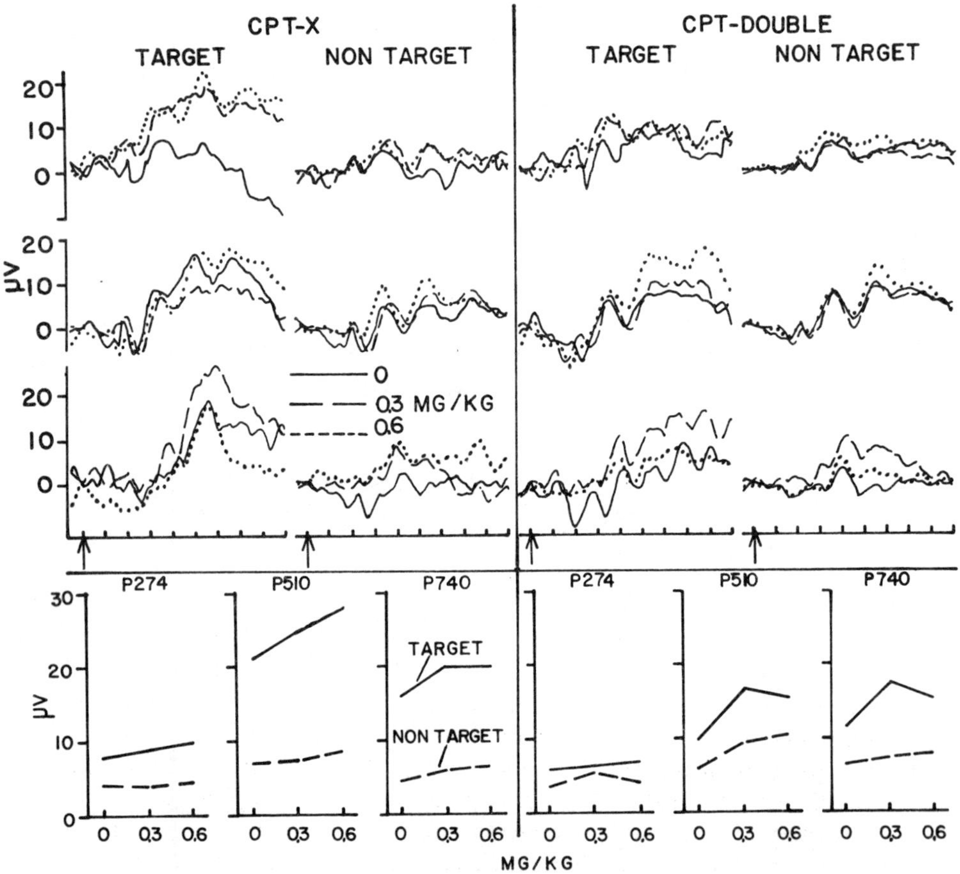

FIG. 4.13 The top panel depicts three cross-situational ADD patients' ERP waveforms under each pharmacologic condition. Positive amplitudes at the parietal electrodes are depicted upward. Stimulus onset is marked by an arrow and the abscissa is demarcated in intervals of 100-msec. The lower panel displays mean amplitude for the cross-situational group for three components of the late positive complex. For P510 and P740, the two doses of methylphenidate yielded comparable increases in amplitude of P510 and P740 in both tasks. (Reproduced from Klorman *et al.* [1983] with permission of Elsevier Scientific Publishers, Ireland.)

exclusive reliance on either of these tasks could lead to erroneous conclusions about pharmacologic effects.

Results: ERP

The top panel of Figure 4.13 displays three illustrative individual ERP waveforms for each task and dosage. Average amplitudes for three positive peaks (mean latencies = 274, 510, and 740 milliseconds post-stimulus, respectively) in the late positive complex are depicted in the lower panel. All three peaks showed larger amplitude in response to targets than nontargets, i.e., reflected task requirements. However, only the later two peaks were affected by stimulant medication. In both instances, the two doses of methylphenidate comparably increased ERP amplitude over placebo levels ($p < 0.0001$). Once again, there were no differences between the cross situational and borderline ADD samples.

Some comment is required by the similarity of findings for the two late positive peaks. One should not infer that this result implies nonspecific changes in arousal, rather than in attention. As emphasized in the discussion section of Clinical Challenge, Study 2, there is weak or contradictory evidence that stimulant medication consistently augments LPC amplitude to visual stimuli in tasks without active attentional demands. Present knowledge indicates that the various LPC waves reflect different aspects of cognitive processing. Yet, although all three peaks reflected the attentional aspects of the task, only the latter two were affected by methylphenidate. These results suggest some specificity in the cognitive processes augmented by this stimulant drug.

Discussion

Overall, the results of this study were remarkably consistent for the two doses and samples. Comparable enhancement of placebo levels of performance and concomitant ERP amplitude was obtained for the two doses. As a general rule, doubling the strength of the lower dose did not increase the resulting cognitive gains. As noted earlier, Sprague and his colleagues repeatedly have made this observation with a memory test, noting that still higher doses (i.e., 1 mg/kg) impaired performance. Of course, in the present study there were individual differences that were masked by group results. Patients varied with regard to which dose was optimal for them. In fact, the results tend to show a slight, but nonsignificant advantage for the higher dose.

The similarity of results for the cross-situational and borderline samples has important implications for clinical practice. First, of course, one might question this diagnostic distinction. A skeptic might attribute the borderline patients' failure to meet our research criteria to reticence on the part of either teacher or parent. Notably, 57% of the borderline patients would have been classified as normal by either their parents' or teachers' ratings, i.e., their scores placed them within a one standard deviation interval above the mean of normal children on either the parent or teacher scale. Although skepticism concerning new diagnostic distinctions is undoubtedly healthy, there are several reasons for taking the "borderline" ADD designation seriously.

Certainly, one must acknowledge the limitations of exclusive reliance on teacher and parent questionnaires for diagnostic classification (Conners and Taylor, 1980, p 930). However, if one accepts high questionnaire scores as valid research criteria for defining ADD, then equal credence should be placed on the significance of borderline scores or discrepancies between teachers' and parents' descriptions of patients. On average, the "borderline" patients' questionnaire scores were considerably elevated. Indeed, they all warranted referral to a practitioner specializing in children's behavioral disorders. Our contention is that there are a significant number of children who display attentional difficulties but who may fall short of the classic profile of the ADD child. That their borderline ADD status may be due to unreliable descriptions by teachers or parents is beside the point. The point is that the present results suggest that stimulant therapy should be considered for these patients.

WORK IN PROGRESS

Introduction

In recent and ongoing work, we have turned from testing patients after a single administration of medication to conducting clinical trials. The main reason for this change stems from the interest of physicians and parents in determining whether stimulant medication is beneficial for a particular child. Intuitively it seemed more promising to rely on observations drawn after a patient has been exposed to medication for several days, such that he or she has adapted to side effects or dosage has been titrated optimally.

Clinical Studies

One study currently under analysis included 70 patients who participated in a blind clinical trial comprising two counterbalanced phases of 14 days each on methylphenidate (0.3 mg/kg, twice daily) and Placebo. This project was undertaken in collaboration with Dr. Stuart Loeb, Dr. Margaret McBride, and Ms. Jaine Strauss. Patients participated in three sessions held, respectively, before the trial and immediately after receiving their last noon dose for each phase. At each testing, two versions of CPT were administered while concomitant ERPs were measured.

A major purpose of this research was to follow up on recent suggestions (Loney and Millich, 1982; Prinz *et al.*, 1981) that the ADD syndrome comprises inattentive as well as aggressive behaviors. Our initial analyses have disclosed a reduction in rated inattentiveness and aggression with methylphenidate for both inattentive ADD patients and patients combining inattentiveness and aggression. There is also preliminary evidence that both groups of patients profited from stimulant therapy in their performance and ERP during CPT.

A similarly designed clinical study involves a follow-up of ADD patients who have reached adolescence. This work is part of a doctoral dissertation conducted by Ms. Hilary Coons. Thus far, 18 such patients have been tested and the results disclose clinical improvement in the methylphenidate phase of the trial. In addition, in the active phase of the trial, these patients exhibited previously observed gains in performance and LPC amplitude in CPT Double.

Discussion

These results disclose that CPT performance and ERP measures are sensitive not only to acute challenges but also to clinical trials of methylphenidate. Ongoing analyses are aimed at evaluating the practical utility of this work for supplementing other measures of clinical outcome of stimulant therapy. From a theoretical standpoint, it is certainly instructive to establish that designated subsets of the ADD syndrome, e.g., borderline, aggressive, or adolescent patients, as a group, display the characteristic stimulant-induced gains in measures of cognitive functioning. It remains to be established whether these observations provide useful information beyond that available from clinical ratings (Otto *et al.*, 1984). Of course, even if such incremental validity could not be established, there is practical value to the availability of objective techniques for evaluating clinical outcome of therapy when teachers or parents are unavailable or incapable of aiding in such evaluation.

However, the most likely contribution of this approach lies in a different area. Current theorizing and empirical efforts implicate ERPs in specific aspects of cognitive processing. It follows that the most instructive application of ERP or other methodologies to the study of ADD would be to pinpoint *specific* aspects of cognitive function that are impaired in this syndrome or benefit from pharmacotherapy. Rosenthal and Allen (1978) and Sergeant (chapter 1) have emphasized the need for going beyond demonstrations of nonspecific cognitive disturbances, e.g., slow speed or high inaccuracy.

ERP research can aid in bridging these gaps in our knowledge. An initial step has been to extrapolate from research bearing on the cognitive processes associated with specific ERP components. For instance, other laboratories have examined the early negative peak (N1 or N100) held by Hillyard (Hillyard *et al.*, 1978) to reflect early gating of relevant informational channels. In this context, it is especially interesting that Stamm and colleagues found that N100 during dichotic listening tasks was abnormally attenuated in ADD youngsters (Loiselle *et al.*, 1980; Zambelli *et al.*, 1977). Similarly instructive is the demonstration by Halliday and his colleagues that, in a similar discrimination test, methylphenidate increased N100 amplitude in clinical responders to this drug while decreasing its amplitude in nonresponders (Halliday *et al.*, 1976; Halliday *et al.*, 1984). These results illustrate how ERP measures can aid in the identification of specific cognitive aspects of ADD.

Reports from our laboratory as well as others (Loiselle *et al.*, 1980; Prichep *et al.*, 1976; Holcomb and Dykman, 1983) have pointed to abnormally small LPC amplitude in ADD patients during detection tests and the amplification of LPC in these children after methylphenidate. Reference to the literature on LPC shows that the amplitude of these components is sensitive to cognitive capacity allocated to evaluation processes.

A still more informative approach involves the use of experimental paradigms that directly—rather than by inference from other results—implicate the psychological processes held to be impaired in these patients. An illustration of this strategy is presented in Sergeant's chapter in this volume (see chapter 1). In this work, several levels of memory load were studied during search processes and reaction time examined as a measure of processing. We are currently using similar paradigms, in which reaction time as well as the amplitude and latency of LPC are examined in ADD patients subjected to clinical trials of methylphenidate and tested under a range of memory requirements. We believe that this strategy has the potential of aiding in delineating the sources of the ADD child's slowness in such tasks. Specifically, the present work is aimed at determining whether these disturbances involve processes that occur before or after stimuli are evaluated. Similar questions can be examined with regard to the locus of the positive effects of stimulants on reaction time in these procedures.

Further advances in our understanding of ERP processes can suggest experimental designs capitalizing on components reflecting a range of cognitive processes relevant to ADD. This strategy has great potential for further understanding the ADD syndrome and therapeutic interventions for this disorder.

DISCUSSION: SUMMARY

The question was raised as to the connection between the Late Positive Component and P300. These are essentially synonymous terms. P300 was used to designate a positive peak with latency of approximately 300 msec. However, as task complexity increases, this peak's latency may be considerably longer.

One participant noted that in the third challenge study with young adults, methylphenidate affected P464 latencies of targets, not nontargets (Figure 4.11). It is unclear at present whether this result is due to measurement problems or whether it reflects differential processing of targets and nontargets. Some caution is required because this result has not been replicated.

Another participant commented that although a stimulant may have theoretically consistent effects on different measures, different subjects carry these effects for the several variables. The same is the case for the results reported in this chapter.

There was a question about the use of fixed doses rather than individually titrated doses. This choice seemed preferable to the variability that would have resulted if each of the several physicians involved in this project followed his/her preferred approach.

Another question concerned whether the evoked potentials were computed separately for trials on which the subject made correct and incorrect responses. In most of the early studies reported in this chapter, this distinction was not observed because of technical difficulties. In recent work, we have computed ERPs for only correctly identified targets and nontargets. Thus, the findings reported are not attributable to lumping together correctly and incorrectly processed stimuli.

Another participant referred to a study by Yellen (Yellen *et al.*, 1983) in which two types of vigilance tasks are used, which presumably differentiate between two types of patients. If the target is more frequent than the nontarget, the task measures failures of inhibition. When the target is more rare, the task reflects sustained attention. The tasks on which our work is based were all of the latter type. The rate of targets, depending on the study, was 10% to 15%

ACKNOWLEDGMENTS

The research described in this chapter was supported in large part by a contract from the New York State Research Council and Grant MH-32103 from NIMH to the first author. This work benefited greatly from the contributions of the following students and research assistants: Lance Bauer, Joan Brumaghim, Karen Dainer, Hilary Coons, Robin Michael, Hellen Pollack, and Jaine Strauss. We are grateful to Lewis Bloomingdale, Joan Brumaghim, Susan Garnsey, Rhonda Klorman, Joseph Sergeant, and Jaine Strauss for their comments on an earlier draft of this paper.

GENERAL DISCUSSION

Dr. Quay: Is the component you are measuring the same as that referred to in the literature as P300?

Dr. Klorman: Yes. In early experiments P300 peaked at 300 msec; hence the name. However, latency shifts with the complexity of the task and the peak can occur at 600 msec or longer. Consequently, I call it the late positive component. In the present study, I assigned to it its mean latency.

Dr. Quay: Is it possible to determine whether your subjects are augmenters or reducers over time?

Dr. Klorman: To do that I would have to run a different series. We did report data on that question in a double-dose study (Klorman *et al.*, 1983).

Dr. Ferguson: When you looked at increases in latency in the older group on placebo, you showed large increases in latency for the targets but no increases in latency for nontargets. Does that mean that people do not process nontargets? Also, you showed a slide in which components peaked at a little over either 200, 500 or 700 msec with slight differences in magnitude.

Dr. Klorman: I don't know why the latency for nontargets does not change. On the second point, you are referring to data on 0, 0.3 and 0.6 mg/kg doses where we scored different components. It is true that evoked responses produce multiple positive peaks and many are sensitive to attention. While there is some controversy about the precise meaning of all of those peaks, there is most agreement about the meaning of the middle component. Since the response to nontargets was smaller, peaks were more difficult to identify.

Dr. Pelham: You are giving mean differences on all variables. When we did that with behavioral data, we found that although there are mean differences in all measures, different subjects account for the effects in different means.

Dr. Klorman: I haven't run correlations recently but what you say is true. Different subjects do account for the trends on different measures.

Dr. Simeon: Why did you use a fixed rather than a therapeutic dose of Ritalin? Also, is the drug-induced increase in evoked potential due to the CPT experimental procedure? That is, are there differences between errors of omission and errors of commission?

Dr. Klorman: I used a fixed dose because I'm not a physician. I study patients referred by different physicians, each with a different practice and using different criteria for titration. Variable doses would have added noise to the experiment. As to errors of omission and commission on the CPT, I recently tried to look only at evoked response when the subject made what was an appropriate response—a hit, not an omission or a false alarm.

Dr. Simeon: With medication, both type of errors, omission and commission, decreased. When you looked at evoked potential, you combined both responses.

Dr. Klorman: We have only been looking at those instances when the subject didn't make an error, so that the effects of amplitude are not an artifact combining the two kinds of trials.

Dr. Sergeant: Were the differences between target and nontarget measurements significant with respect to placebo and MPD?

Dr. Klorman: Probably not.

Dr. Sergeant: If a drug influences responses both to the target and to nontargets, in all probability a generalized arousability factor is being influenced. Have you considered that the arousability of the subjects rather than stimulus evaluation is being influenced; i.e., the phase at responding is changing equally for the target and nontarget?

Dr. Klorman: The situation is not one in which you tell a subject to count tones and ignore flashes. Technically, our experiment is an excessive discrimination task. The subject has to pay a great deal of attention to nontargets; they enable him to know the targets. Failure to find increasing differences between targets and nontargets with medication does not address the question of selective attention.

Dr. Hechtman: Yellen (Yellen *et al.*, 1983) proposed a concept that perhaps what we call ADD could really be divided into two subgroups. One group is the children who have difficulty inhibiting responses; they are primarily impulsive children. The other children have more problems with sustained attention but are not as impulsive. This is reflected in the difference in errors of omission and errors of commission. Yellen suggested the frequency of the stimulus presentation differentiates between these two groups. With a frequent stimulus presentation, the task is really to inhibit the response to the nonrelevant stimulus. Where you have an infrequent stimulus presentation, the task is to respond correctly. What was the frequency of stimulus presentation in your study and what are your thoughts about the subgroup with the particular problem type you measured?

Dr. Klorman: The frequency of presentation was what probably would be called frequent, i.e., every second and one-half, for two reasons: (a) the child can only be in testing just so long, doing both potentials where a lot of trials can be obtained, and (b) it is the frequency used most often in the

ADD literature. It is the order of frequency sensitive to changes in vigilance. Errors of commission have a very different meaning in a single than in a double task, where you must attend to the previous trial or you don't know what this one means, like the X task. The process involved would be different. In terms of distinction per se, I can't give a definitive answer at this time.

Dr. Hechtman: I guess Dr. Yellen's point was that the absolute frequency was not as important as whether the subject responds most of the time and has a response set. It's the ratio of stimuli to which the subject must respond vs. the ratio of stimuli to which the subject does not have to respond.

Dr. Klorman: Depending on the experiment, 10% to 15% were targets in our study.

Dr. Sergeant: We are dealing with CPT tasks in which the event rate is as important a variable as the ratio between target and nontarget. We built in, automatically, 10% for the CPT, so there is a great tendency to miss the target. The critical point about new types of continuous tasks is that it puts the load on short-term memory processes, whereas the older CPT tested vigilance only.

Dr. Hunt: Comparing the double CPT task to the single, is there a delay in the positive component, or an increase in the latency of response?

Dr. Klorman: I have never studied that systematically using the more sensitive measurements we have today. The task turns out to be too easy for college students in the sense that there is a floor effect. We don't get a drug effect, either in performance or on the evoked response, and yet with older subjects it is easiest to identify a peak. We are now using more sophisticated measurement techniques, so I'll be able to answer that question. But, in general, others have shown that the more complex the discrimination, or the longer it takes to make a discrimination in terms of response or reaction time, the later the component peak.

REFERENCES

Aman MG: Drugs, learning and the psychotherapies. In Werry (ed): Pediatric Psychopharmacology. New York, Brunner/Mazel, 1978, pp 79–108.

Chapman LJ, Chapman JP: Problems in the measurement of cognitive deficit. Psychol Bull 1973: 79:380–385.

Conners CK: Ratings scales for use in drug studies with children. In Guy (ed): ECDEU Assessment Manual. Rockville, MD, US Department of Health, Education, and Welfare, 1976, pp 303–312.

Conners CK, Taylor E: Pemoline, methylphenidate and placebo in children with minimal brain dysfunction. Arch Gen Psychiat 1980; 37:922–930.

Conners CK, Werry JS: Pharmacotherapy. In Quay HC and Werry JS (eds): Psychopathological Disorders in Children, 2nd ed. New York; Wiley, 1979, pp 336–386.

Coons HW, Peloquin LJ, Klorman R, Ryan RM, Bauer LO, Perlmutter RA, Salzman LF: Effects of methylphenidate on young adults' event-related potentials. Electroencephal Clin Neurophysiol 1981; 51:373–387.

Davies DR, Parasuraman R: The Psychology of Vigilance. New York, Academic Press, 1981.

Donchin E, McCarthy G: Event-related brain potentials in the study of cognitive processes. In Ludlow and Doran-Quine (eds): The Neurological Bases of Language Disorders in Children: Methods and Directions for Research. Bethesda, US Department of Health, Education, and Welfare, 1979, pp 109–128.

Friedman D, Vaughan HG, Erlenmeyer-Kimling L: Multiple late positive potentials in two visual discrimination tasks. Psychophysiology 1981; 18:635–649.

Friedman D, Vaughan H, Erlenmeyer-Kimling L: Task-related cortical potentials in children in two kinds of vigilance tasks. In DA Otto (ed): Multidisciplinary perspectives in event-related brain potential research. Washington, DC, US Government Printing Office, 1978, pp 309–313.

Grier JB: Nonparametric indexes for sensitivity and bias: computing formulas Psychol Bull 1971; 75:424–429.

Halliday R, Callaway E, Rosenthal JH: The visual ERP predicts clinical response to methylphenidate in hyperactive children. Psychophysiology 1984; 21:114–121.

Halliday R, Rosenthal JH, Naylor H, Callaway E: Averaged evoked potential predictors of clinical improvement in hyperactive children treated with methylphenidate: An initial study and a replication. Psychophysiology 1976; 13:429–440.

Hillyard SA, Picton TW, Regan D: Sensation, perception, and attention: Analysis using ERPs. In E Callaway, P Tueting and SH Koslow (eds): Event-related Brain Potentials in Man. New York, Academic Press, 1978, pp 223–322.

Holcomb PJ, Dykman RA: Late ERP components in ADD, RD, and normal boys. Psychophysiology 1983; 20:446.

Kinsbourne M: Minimal brain dysfunction as a neurodevelopmental lag. Ann NY Acad Sci 1973; 205:268–273.

Klorman R, Bauer LO, Coons HW, Lewis JL, Peloquin LJ, Perlmutter RA, Ryan RM, Salzman LF, Strauss J: Enhancing effects of methylphenidate on normal young adults' cognitive processes. Psychopharmacol Bull 1984; 20:3–9.

Klorman R, Salzman LF, Bauer LO, Coons HW, Borgstedt AD, Halpern WI: Effects of two doses of methylphenidate on cross-situational and borderline hyperactive children's evoked potentials. Electroencephal Clin Neurophysiol 1983; 56:169–185.

Klorman R, Salzman LF, Pass HL, Borgstedt AD, Dainer KB: Effects of methylphenidate on hyperactive children's evoked responses during passive and active attention. Psychophysiology 1979; 16:23–29.

Loiselle D, Stamm JS, Maitinsky S, Whipple SC: Evoked potential and behavioral signs of attentive dysfunctions in hyperactive boys. Psychophysiology 1980; 17:193–201.

Loney J, Milich R: Hyperactivity inattention, and aggression in clinical practice. In Wolraich and Routh (eds): Advances in Developmental and Behavioral Pediatrics, vol 2. Greenwich, Connecticut, JAI Press, 1982; pp 113–147.

Michael RL, Klorman R, Salzman LF, Borgstedt AD, Dainer KB: Normalizing effects of methylphenidate on hyperactive children's vigilance performance and evoked potentials. Psychophysiology 1981; 18:665–677.

O'Dougherty M, Nuechterlein KH, Drew B: Hyperactive and hypoxic children: signal detection, sustained attention and behavior. J Abnorm Psycho 1984; 93:178–191.

Otto D, Karrer R, Halliday R, Horst RL, Klorman R, Squires N, Thatcher RW, Fenelon B, Lelord G: Developmental aspects of event-related potentials: aberrant development. Ann NY Acad Sci 1984; 425:319–337.

Paine RS, Oppe TF: Neurological examination of children. Clin Dev Med 1966; 20/21.

Perel JM, Dayton PG: Methylphenidate. In Usdin and Forrest (eds): Psychotherapeutic drugs. New York, Marcel Dekker, Part II, 1978, pp 1287–1316.

Picton TW, Stuss DT: The component structure of the human event-related potentials. Prog Brain Res 1980; 54:17–49.

Prichep LS, Sutton S, Hakerem G: Evoked potentials in hyperkinetic and normal children under certainty and uncertainty: a placebo and methylphenidate study. Psychophysiology 1976; 13:419–428.

Prinz RN, Connor PA, Wilson CC: Hyperactive and aggressive behaviors in childhood: Intertwined dimensions. J Abnorm Child Psychol 1981; 9:191–202.

Pritchard WS: Psychophysiology of P300. Psychol Bull 1981; 89:506–540.

Rapoport JL, Buchsbaum MS, Weingartner H, Zahn TP, Ludlow C, Bartko J, Mikkelsen EJ, Langer DH, Burney WE: Dextroamphetamine: cognitive and behavioral effects in normal and hyperactive boys and normal adult males. Arch Gen Psychiat 1980; 37:933–943.

Rosenthal RH, Allen TW: Intratask destractibility in hyperkinetic and nonhyperkinetic children. J Abnorm Child Psychol 1980; 8:175–187.

Rosvold HE, Mirsky AF, Sarason I, Bansome ED, Beck LH: A continuous performance test of brain damage. J Consult Psychol 1956; 20:343–350.

Shagass C, Ornitz EM, Sutton S, Tueting P: Event related potentials and psychopathology. In Callaway, Tueting and Koslow (eds): Event Related Potentials in Man. New York, Academic Press, 1978, pp 443–496.

Sostek AJ, Buchsbaum MS, Rapoport JL: Effects of amphetamine on vigilance performance in normal and hyperactive children. J Abnorm Child Psychol 1980; 8:491–500.

Sprague RL, Christensen DE, Werry JS: Experimental psychology and stimulant drugs. In Conners (ed): Clinical Use of Stimulant Drugs in Children. New York, American Elsevier, 1974, pp 141–163.

Sprague RL, Sleator EK: What is the proper dose of stimulant drugs in children? Int J Ment Health 1975; 4:75–104.

Sprague RL, Sleator EK: Methylphenidate in hyperkinetic children: differences in dose effects on learning and social behavior. Science 1977; 198:1274–1276.

Sroufe LA: Drug treatment of children with behavior problems. In Horowitz (ed): Review of child development research. Chicago, University of Chicago Press, 1975, pp 347–407.

Strauss J, Lewis JL, Klorman R, Peloquin LJ, Perlmutter RA, Salzman LF: Effects of methylphenidate on young adults' performance and event related potentials in a vigilance and a paired associates learning test. Psychophysiology 1984; 21:609–661.

Sutton S, Ruchkin DS: The late positive complex-advances and new problems. Address delivered at the Fourth Evoked Potentials International Conference, Lake Forest, IL, June 1981.

Sykes DH, Douglas VI, Weiss G, Minde K: Attention in hyperactive children and the effect of methylphenidate (Ritalin). J Child Psychol Psychiat 1971; 12:129–139.

Weiss B, Laties VG: Enhancement of human performance by caffeine and the amphetamines. Pharmacol Rev 1962; 14:1–36.

Werry JS, Sprague RL: Hyperactivity. In Costello (ed): Symptoms of Psychopathology. New York, Wiley, 1970, pp 397–417.

Werry JS, Sprague RL: Methylphenidate in children—effect of dosage. Aust NZ J Psychiat 1974; 8:9–19.

Yellen AM, Greenberg L, Hopwood J: Inhibition deficit disorder (I.D.D.) evidence supporting differentiation from attention deficit disorder. Presented at the American Academy of Child Psychiatry Annual Meeting, San Francisco, CA October 1983.

Zambelli AJ, Stamm JS, Maitinsky S, Loiselle DL: Auditory evoked potentials in formerly hyperactive adolescents. Am J Psychiat 1977; 134:742–747.

5

The Clinical Importance of Methylphenidate Blood Level Determinations

C. THOMAS GUALTIERI, ROBERT E. HICKS, RANDALL W. EVANS AND KENNERLY PATRICK

INTRODUCTION

In earlier publications, we reported the preliminary findings of a research program concerned with blood levels and the pharmacokinetics of methylphenidate (MPD). On the basis of a highly sensitive and reliable gas chromatographic-mass spectroscopic method for measuring MPD, the pharmacokinetic characteristics of the drug have been described in hyperactive children (HAC, Attention Deficit Disorder with Hyperactivity), hyperactive adults (Attention Deficit Disorder, Residual Type), normal adults, and also in rats and monkeys (Gualtieri *et al.*, 1982a,b; Wargin *et al.*, 1983). These findings were largely in agreement with those reported by other investigators (Hungund *et al.*, 1979; Shaywitz *et al.*, 1982; Winsberg *et al.*, 1982; Chan *et al.*, 1980). The fact that MPD serum levels do not differ when the drug is ingested in the fasting state or after a full meal was reported by our group (Gualtieri *et al.*, 1982a,b) on the basis of a small study conducted in normal adults, and was subsequently confirmed in a study of HAC by Chan *et al.* (1983).

We have also reported, on two occasions, that MPD serum levels did not appear to correlate, to any significant degree, with measures of clinical response. These reports were based on preliminary analyses of data from a double-blind crossover of MPD at two clinically relevant doses (0.3 and 0.6 mg/kg). However, the opinions expressed in those two papers were not confirmed by other investigators. In fact, three recent reports have appeared, maintaining that MPD blood levels (BL) may actually be related to different aspects of the clinical response (Shaywitz *et al.*, 1982; Winsberg *et al.*, 1980, 1982); and even that MPD BL determinations might prove useful in the clinical management of HAC (Shaywitz *et al.*, 1982).

The completed analysis of a series of studies concerned with the clinical utility of MPD serum levels, however, has confirmed our earlier contention that MPD serum levels are not, in fact, related to clinical response or to side effects. Furthermore, it is highly unlikely that MPD serum levels will prove to be clinically important.

Five research studies are described. In two studies, MPD serum levels were correlated with different aspects of the clinical response in a between-groups analysis. These were studied of the acute effects of MPD in 55 HAC subjects and a study of the pharmacokinetic time profile of MPD in 26 HAC subjects. A within-subject analysis was done in two studies of the pharmacokinetic time profile of MPD in 12 HAC and in 10 normal adult volunteers, and, in a third study of the clinical correlations of MPD, serum-level variability in four HAC. A comparison of MPD time profiles in HAC and in normal adult volunteers is also described.

METHODS

The specific details of each study are given below, and clinical data describing subjects are given in Table 5.1.

Subjects

For admission to the clinical studies, HAC subjects were required to meet DSM-III criteria for the diagnosis of Attention Deficit Disorder with Hyperactivity (American Psychiatric Association, 1978), and to score two standard deviations above the mean for sex and age on the hyperactivity and distractibility factors of the Conners Teacher Rating Scale (CTRS) (Goyette *et al.*, 1978). All HAC were drug-naive prior to entry to the studies, unless otherwise specified. Subjects were boys and girls, outpatients and inpatients, whites and blacks, ages 6 to 13, with an IQ

TABLE 5.1 *Classification of subjects in five studies reported*

		Study				
		I	II	III	IV	V
Subjects		HAC	HAC	HAC	NAD	HAC
Analysis		BG	BG	WS	WS	WS
N		55	26	11	10	4
Age (mean)		8.4	9.5	9.0	28.5	6.8
Sex	M	39	22	9	10	3
	F	16	4	2	0	1
Race	W	42	14	10	10	4
	NW	13	2	1	0	0
Inpatients		30	20	9	0	4
Outpatients		25	6	2	10	0

HAC = hyperactive children; NAD = normal adult male volunteers; BG = between groups; WS = within subjects.

above 70, in good general health, and on no intercurrent medications. Parents gave informed consent and children gave their assent to all aspects of the research.

Normal adult male volunteers (age 18–35) were recruited from the university community. All subjects were in good medical and psychologic health, of average height and weight, on no intercurrent medications, and nonsmokers. Normal adults gave informed consent and were reimbursed for time and effort spent in the research protocols.

Blood Level Determinations

Methods of blood collection and MPD analysis have been reported previously (Gualtieri *et al.*, 1982a,b; Wargin *et al.*, 1983). Serum MPD concentrations were determined by the mass fragmentographic method of Patrick *et al.* (1985) using deuterium-enriched MPD as an internal standard (see Patrick *et al.*, 1982 for synthesis). The assay involves a two-step solvent extraction procedure, gas chromatographic separation and selected ion monitoring of the piperidyl fragments of MPD and penta-deuterated MPD as their pentafluoropropionyl derivatives. The within-run coefficient of variation, using this method, was 5.2% (at 1 ng/ml) or 6% (at 9 ng/ml), with a practical limit of detection of 500 pg/ml. To further establish the reliability of the method, blood samples were exchanged with a second laboratory, which has published clinical data on MPD blood levels. This laboratory uses a gas chromatographic method with thermionic specific detection (Jatlow, 1983). Values obtained by the two laboratories were highly correlated ($r = 0.99$).

Blood samples were taken from subjects in standard ways, either through a "butterfly" infusion set inserted into the antecubital vein, or, for subjects who were studied for pharmacokinetic time profiles, through a heparinized indwelling venous catheter. Samples were drawn into a plastic syringe, allowed to clot in a glass tube, spun, separated, and frozen.

All subjects were tested in the early morning, having fasted from midnight, and maintained a pattern of light activity during the study period.

THE ACUTE EFFECTS STUDY (AES)

Subjects

Fifth-five HAC were subjects in this study. Subjects were included if, after a thorough neuropsychiatric evaluation, they met the criteria outlined above. The mean age was 8.4 years; additional descriptive data are given in Tables 5.1 and 5.2. Thirty HAC were inpatients on a child psychiatry service, and 25 were outpatients in a pediatric neuropsychiatry clinic.

TABLE 5.2 *Acute effects study (HAC)*

		Inpatients	Outpatients	Total group
N		30	25	55
Age		8.3 ± 1.8	8.5 ± 2.3	8.4 ± 2.0
Sex	M	17	22	39
	F	13	3	16
SES		3.8 ± 1.4	3.2 ± 1.1	3.5 ± 1.3
PPVT		99.8 ± 16.1	101.4 ± 15.1	100.7 ± 15.4
FSIQ		80.2 ± 20.5	79.0 ± 7.2	80.1 ± 19.5
MPD serum level (0.3 mg/kg)				
$\bar{X} \pm SD$		11.4 ± 5.5	11.1 ± 5.7	11.3 ± 5.5
Range		1.2–24.2	1.4–21.1	1.2–24.2
N		24	24	48
MPD serum level (0.6 mg/kg)				
$\bar{X} \pm SD$		22.8 ± 13.1	24.7 ± 15.6	23.8 ± 14.2
Range		4.3–63.5	2.3–70.1	2.3–70.1
N		25	23	48

SES = Socio-economic status (Hollingshead-Redlich); PPVT = Peabody Picture Vocabulary Test; FSIQ = Full Scale IQ, WISC-R or Stanford-Binet.

Although inpatients tended to have more severe conditions and came from less-advantaged families, there were no other important differences between the two groups (Table 5.2).

Method

There were three experimental conditions, following baseline evaluation: placebo, and MPD in two doses, 0.3 and 0.6 mg/kg/dose. The conditions were counterbalanced and randomly assigned, and the study was double-blind. Drug or placebo was administered on a b.i.d. basis, at 8 a.m. and 12 noon.

On the first day of each condition, the first dose was administered in the clinic by a research nurse. Pulse and blood pressure were measured in the supine position. An hour later, a venous blood sample was drawn for MPD SL, growth hormone, prolactin, and thyroid-stimulating hormone (by radioimmune assay). Then the subject was administered a battery of tests that were time-locked to the time of medication administration. These were: the Continuous Performance Task (CPT) (Rosvold *et al.*, 1956) with a wrist-watch actometer on the subject's nondominant arm: the Kagan Matching Familiar Figures Test (Egeland, 1976); and a 15-minute session in a free-field laboratory playroom (Routh Activity Room, RAR) (Routh *et al.*, 1974).

All subsequent medication was administered orally by parents (outpatients) or nurses (inpatients). At the end of each week, parents (outpatients) or nurses (inpatients) and teachers would complete the abbreviated CTRS and a side-effect checklist. Classroom behavior was measured by research assistants and teachers using an interval behavior observation system (Wahler *et al.*, 1976). At the end of each condition, the global impressions of parents (or nurses) and teachers were solicited directly or by telephone.

Global response was rated on a three-point scale: 1 = improved; 2 = minimal change; 3 = no change or worse on drug. Side effects were rated as absent, mild, moderate or severe. Total response incorporated changes in three areas: global response, side effects, and degree of change in the CTRS. Total response was rated on a 1 to 5 basis, according to the following algorithm:

TR = 1 (Best responders). Global = 1; side effects absent or mild; CTRS change more than 2 *SD* for age and sex for total score, hyperactivity and distractibility factors; decision to continue drug after study.

TR = 2 Global = 1; side effects absent or mild; CTRS changes more than 1 *SD*; decision to continue drug.

TR = 3 Global = 1; side effects absent or mild; improvement on CTRS, but less than 1 *SD*; decision to continue drug.

TR = 4 Global = 2; side effects absent or mild; decision to continue drug for a while longer to evaluate response.

TR = 5 (Poorest responders). Global = 3; decision not to continue MPD.

Analysis, Results

MPD serum levels did not differ among the five total response categories, or among the four side effect categories, at either dose (Table 5.3 and 5.4). At the 0.3-mg/kg dose, MPD serum levels at 1 hour did not correlate

TABLE 5.3 *Methylphenidate serum levels at different clinical levels of response*

Total response	Methylphenidate serum levels (ng/ml)		
	$(\bar{X} \pm SD)$	Range	*N*
Low dose (0.3 mg/kg)			
1 (best)	7.7 ± 3.0	5.9–11.2	3
2	13.5 ± 6.1	4.2–24.2	9
3	10.4 ± 5.7	1.4–19.7	12
4	13.5 ± 6.4	5.1–21.1	10
5 (poorest)	9.7 ± 4.1	1.2–16.4	14
High dose (0.6 mg/kg)			
1 (best)	12.9 ± 12.7	3.9–21.8	2
2	24.2 ± 16.7	2.3–57.8	11
3	27.1 ± 16.1	12.2–70.1	11
4	26.9 ± 14.9	4.3–63.5	11
5 (poorest)	19.5 ± 9.3	4.4–33.7	13

TABLE 5.4 *Methylphenidate serum levels and side effects*

Side effects	Serum levels (ng/ml) $\bar{X} \pm SD$	Range	*N*
Low dose (0.3 mg/kg)			
None	11.2 ± 5.6	1.2–24.2	36
Mild	12.1 ± 5.5	1.4–19.7	10
Moderate	8.6 ± 4.9	5.1–12.0	2
Severe	—	—	0
High dose (0.6 mg/kg)			
None	22.0 ± 17.1	2.3–70.1	23
Mild	21.3 ± 9.3	5.1–39.7	11
Moderate	29.3 ± 14.3	17.9–63.5	8
Severe	27.6 ± 7.6	16.1–36.3	6

with total response category ($r = -0.06$, Pearson Product Moment Correlation), global response ($r = -0.10$), side effects category ($r = -0.01$), change in CTRS score in absolute terms ($r = 0.13$), or in terms of standard deviations ($r = 0.15$), change in the CTRS hyperactivity items ($r = 0.21$) [absolute], $r = 0.24$ [relative to norms], or change in CTRS distractibility

TABLE 5.5 *Correlations of Methylphenidate serum levels and response measures*

Dependent measure	Dose Methylphenidate (mg/kg) 0.3 mg/kg *N*	*R*	0.6 mg/kg *N*	*R*
Conners Parent Rating Scale				
Total score	40	−0.104	39	−0.080
Hyperactivity items	39	−0.136	37	0.012
Distractibility items	39	−0.049	36	−0.065
Conners Teacher Rating Scale				
Total score	26	−0.237	23	0.319
Hyperactivity items	23	−0.220	21	0.027
Distractibility items			20	0.324
Pulse rate	31	0.311	33	0.370*
Systolic blood pressure	31	0.395*	33	0.178
Diastolic blood pressure	29	0.479*	32	0.248
Growth hormone	39	0.318	40	0.207
Prolactin	33	−0.062	34	0.291
Thyroid stimulating hormone	14	−0.361	14	−0.148
Continuous performance task				
Correct responses	36	0.109	37	−0.043
False alarms	34	−0.215	36	−0.210
Actometer	33	−0.061	34	−0.194
Matching familiar figures				
Latency	28	−0.139	28	0.104
Errors	27	−0.344	26	−0.309
Routh Activity Room				
Quadrant entries	38	0.133	35	0.317
Toy changes	38	0.004	38	0.128

TABLE 5.5—*Continued*

Dependent measure	Dose Methylphenidate (mg/kg)			
	0.3 mg/kg		0.6 mg/kg	
	N	*R*	*N*	*R*
Behavioral observations by research assistant				
3	11	−0.300	14	−0.224
4	10	−0.384	13	−0.169
5	17	0.039	11	0.110
6	12	0.199	12	−0.203
9	1	0.375	10	0.055
10	27	0.088	26	−0.144
12	14	0.596	10	−0.161
13	23	0.050	20	0.091
14	13	−0.604*	10	0.315
15	17	−0.037	16	−0.308
16	5	−0.224	8	0.027
17	25	−0.244	22	−0.132
18	5	−0.302	10	0.328
19	7	0.310	5	−0.112
20	6	−0.153	7	−0.286
21	25	−0.162	23	−0.101
22	22	−0.027	18	0.029
23	5	0.758		
24	4	−0.965		
25	6	−0.251	10	0.489
Behavior observations by Teacher				
1	3	−0.715		
2	12	0.078	8	−0.267
3	9	−0.005	6	−0.041
4	3	0.931	3	0.321
5	5	0.652	6	−0.082
6	4	−0.146		
7	11	0.148	11	0.381
8	13	0.045	11	0.399
9	12	−0.039	11	−0.204

* Significant at $p = 0.05$ level.

items ($r = -0.02$ [absolute], $r = -0.03$ [relative]). At the 0.6-mg/kg dose, MPD serum levels did not correlate with total response category ($r = -0.05$), global response (-0.02), occurence of side effects ($r = 0.18$), CTRS change ($r = -0.13$ [absolute], $r = -0.09$ [relative], hyperactivity items ($r = 0.05$ [absolute], $r = 0.11$ [relative]) or distractibility items ($r = -0.27$ [absolute], $r = -0.31$ [relative]).

Additional analyses were performed to determine whether MPD serum levels at either dose correlated with specific, rather than global estimates of drug response. In this analysis, dependent measures included changes in the Conners Parent and Teacher Rating Scales, laboratory measures of attention and activity, pulse, blood pressure, growth hormone and prolactin, and direct behavior observations in the classroom. Response on each dependent measure at low and high doses was computed as log (response score on drug/response score on placebo). Each derived function was correlated with log (MPD serum level) at that dose, and the results are given in Table 5.5. Of 91 correlation coefficients listed in the table, only 4 are significant at the 0.05 level, exactly as would be predicted on the basis of chance alone.

CLINICAL CORRELATES OF PHARMACOKINETIC PROFILE IN HAC

Subjects, Methods

Of 55 children who participated in the acute effects study, 26 underwent an MPD pharmacokinetic time profile analysis prior to entry into the study. About 1 week before the acute effects study, a pharmacokinetic time profile was drawn over 8 hours after a 0.3-mg/kg dose of MPD. Bloods were drawn through an indwelling venous catheter at 0, 30, 60, 90, 120, 240, 360 and 480 minutes after the oral dose. The subjects then pursued a pattern of light activity under close supervision during the day.

Various parameters of the pharmacokinetic time profile were then derived, and related to the child's response to MPD during the subsequent acute effects study. These were: 1-hour serum levels of MPD, peak MPD levels, time to peak, MPD half-life, and area under the pharmacokinetic curve (AUC). The dependent measures were salient clinical response measures taken during the low-dose condition of the acute effects study; total response, presence and severity of side effects; change from placebo in the CTRS total score; and in the hyperactivity and distractibility items thereof. Changes in CTRS scores were measured in absolute terms, and also relative to published norms for age and sex (Goyette *et al.*, 1978).

Analysis, Results

The pharmacokinetic parameters are given in Table 5.6. A correlation matrix was derived (Pearson's Product Moment Correlation), including all

TABLE 5.6 *Pharmacokinetic parameters of MPD (0.3 mg/kg) (26 HAC, Study II)*

	Mean ± standard deviation
Half life (hr) ($T\frac{1}{2}$)	2.4 ± 0.6
Time to peak (min) (TTP)	103.8 ± 52.5
MPD serum level peak (ng/ml) (SLP)	12.6 ± 12.2
MPD 1-hr serum level (ng/ml) (SLI)	9.1 ± 4.6
Area under curve (AUC)	3026.9 ± 2930.2

TABLE 5.7 *Clinical response correlations with pharmacokinetic parameters*

	$T\frac{1}{2}$[a]	TTP[b]	SLP[c]	SLI[d]	AUC[e]
Age	0.18	0.00	0.04	−0.28	−0.02
Race	−0.26	−0.32	0.07	0.23	0.00
Sex	0.30	0.20	−0.01	−0.32	0.09
Side	0.03	0.06	0.02	0.08	0.13
TDF	−0.27	−0.01	0.00	0.06	0.00
HDF	−0.52*	0.12	−0.16	0.15	−0.08
DDF	−0.20	−0.14	−0.15	−0.10	−0.09
TSD	−0.24	−0.03	−0.02	0.07	−0.03
HSD	−0.47*	0.18	−0.20	0.07	−0.13
DSD	−0.15	−0.15	−0.27	−0.13	−0.20
Global	0.31	−0.12	0.17	0.37	0.24

[a] $T\frac{1}{2}$ = half life; [b]TTP = time to peak; [c]SLP = MPD SL at peak; [d]SLI = MPD SL at 1 hr; [e]AUC = area under the curve.

* $p < 0.05$; with 55 correlations, two or three will be significant at the 0.05 level on the basis of chance alone.

of the measures described above. The only significant correlations occurred among the pharmacokinetic variables (e.g., between 1 hour MPD and the AUC, $r = 0.47$, $p = 0.05$; peak MPD serum levels and AUC, $r = 0.96$, $p < 0.001$) or among clinical response measures (e.g., between "global" response and decrease in score in the abbreviated CTRS, $r = -0.68$, $p < 0.01$). No significant correlations were found between pharmacokinetic variables and any of the clinical response measures (See Table 5.7).

NEUROENDOCRINE CORRELATES OF MPD SERUM LEVELS AND PHARMACOKINETIC TIME PROFILE (HAC)

Subjects, Methods

In 11 of the 26 HAC in Study 2, assays of the anterior pituitary growth hormones (GH) and prolactin (PRL) were made along the pharmacokinetic time profile of MPD, dose 0.3 mg/kg.

Analysis, Results

Within subjects, autocorrelations were done between MPD serum levels, GH and PRL at seven time points following drug administration. The mean autocorrelations were obtained by Fischer's r to z transformation. The mean correlation between MPD and GH was not significant ($r = 0.54$, $p > 0.05$) while the correlation between MPD and PRL was significant at the $p = 0.05$ level ($r = 0.68$).

Because the correlation between MPD serum level and PRL, in the absence of a placebo group, may have been a function of shared trends rather than actual association, a de-trended analysis (Ostrom, 1978) was performed in the 4 (of 11) individuals for whom the autocorrelation coefficients were significant at the 0.05 level. Once the MPD serum and PRL levels were de-trended, however, the correlations were no longer significant.

NEUROENDOCRINE AND MOOD CORRELATES OF MPD SERUM LEVELS AND PHARMACOKINETIC TIME PROFILE (NORMAL VOLUNTEERS)

Subjects, Method

MPD pharmacokinetic time profiles were measured in ten normal adult volunteers following an oral dose of MPD. Five subjects received MPD at two dose levels, 0.15 and 0.30 mg/kg, as well as identical placebo. Five subjects received only the 0.3-mg/kg dose of MPD and placebo. Doses were randomly assigned, counter-balanced and double-blind. Test days were separated, in each subject, by at least 1 week. GH and PRL levels in serum were also assayed, and pulse and blood pressure were recorded along the course of the curve. Before drug administration, and immediately prior to each blood sample, subjects estimated their overall mood level on a 100-mm linear scale.

Analysis, Results

The data were analyzed in several ways. First, each variable was subjected to a split-plot analysis-of-variance with dosage (placebo, 0.15 mg/kg, and 0.3 mg/kg) as a between-subject factor, and measurement time as a within-subject factor. Main effects and interactions were decomposed using orthogonal polynomial analysis with explicit deviation-from-fit error terms (Grant, 1956) to avoid possible complications of nonsphericity. The weighting coefficients for the measurement-time factor were based on the logarithms of the time intervals to reflect the roughly logarithmic spacing. The unequal interval problem was solved with the Gaito (1973) procedure. These analyses were intended to assess drug responsivity and level of response for each variable across time.

Second, an autocorrelation was obtained for each subject on each pair of variables. The autocorrelations were then subjected to analysis-of-variance with dosage as a grouping variable. These analyses were undertaken to measure the extent to which the variables covaried within subjects across time, and whether the covariance was a function of drug dosage.

Analyses of Variance

MPD Serum level

This variable was recorded in nanograms per milliliter (ng/ml). The 0.3 mg/kg group mean (4.36) differed from the 0.15 mg/kg group mean (2.1), $F(1,9) = 16.19$, $p = 0.003$. The group difference is not constant across time intervals, however, as reflected in the time × dosage interaction, $F(9,81) = 2.14$, $p = 0.35$. This interaction is due to the higher asymptote of the 0.3 group; i.e., dosage × time quadratic, $F(1,9) = 5.56$, $p = 0.43$, is the only significant component.

The main effect of time is significant, $F(9,81) = 21.49$, $p < 0.00001$. The decomposition of this effect reveals significant linear [$F(1,9) = 31.23$, $p = 0.003$] quadratic [$F(1,9) = 14.07$, $p = 0.0045$], and cubic [$F(1,9) = 80.29$, $p = 0.00001$] components.

Growth Hormone

The mean levels of this variable (GH, in ng/ml) are 18.86, 13.7, and 26.29 for the placebo, 0.15-mg/kg and 0.3-mg/kg groups. These apparent differences were not significant statistically, ($p > 0.1$ for the main effect and both components.) There is a dosage × time quadratic interaction, $F(2,17) = 3.61$, $p < 0.05$. This interaction reflects the higher peak of the 0.3-group as compared to the other two groups; 0.3-mg/kg groups vs. (0.15-mg/kg group + placebo) × time quadratic, $F(1,17) = 6.15$, $p < 0.05$. The latter two groups do not differ on the quadratic component of time, $F > 1.0$.

Prolactin

The mean level (ng/ml) of this variable (PRL) are 6.3, 7.9, and 6.0 for the placebo, the 0.15-mg/kg and the 0.3-mg/kg group, $F(2,17) = 1.97$, $p > 0.1$. The dosage × time interaction and all its components fail to reach statistical significance, $p > 0.1$.

The time main effect is significant, $F(9,153) = 11.77$, $p < 0.00001$. The apparent decline in level of response across time is significant: time linear, $F(1,17) = 7.09$, $p = 0.016$, as is the positive trend after about 3 hours; time quadratic, $F(1,17) = 35.63$, $p < 0.00001$. The significant cubic component $F(1,17) = 43.24$, $p < 0.00001$ reflects the shallower slope in the decline of the function through 2 hours (slope = −12.3 log time) as compared to the increasing portion of the function beginning at 3 hours (slope = +33 log time).

Mood

The overall trend for mood responses is an increase in positivity through the first 2 hours, followed by a decline during the last 6 hours; time quadratic, $F(1,11) = 18.62$, $p = 0.001$. However, the significant dosage × time quadratic interaction [$F(2,11) = 9.26$, $p = 0.004$] indicates differences in trend across groups. The interaction further decomposes into dosage linear × time quadratic, $F(1,11) = 13.07$, $p < 0.001$, and is easily described: The placebo group shows a decline through the first 2 hours followed by a recovery, whereas the two drug groups show an increase across the first 2 hours followed by a decline. Among the drug groups, this trend is more accentuated in the 0.3 mg/kg group.

Systolic Blood Pressure

The only significant effect on systolic blood pressure is the quadratic component of time, $F(1,11) = 6.93$, $P = 0.02$.

Diastolic Blood Pressure

There are no significant effects on diastolic blood pressure.

Pulse

There is a significant time effect [$F(9,99) = 3.5$, $p = 0.0008$] composed of linear [$F(1,11) = 7.07$, $p = 0.02$] and quadratic [$F(1,11) = 10.54$, $p = 0.008$] components on pulse rate.

Autocorrelations

The mean autocorrelations area presented in Table 5.8. None of the correlations is significant for the placebo group.

TABLE 5.8 *Correlations with serum levels along pharmacokinetic curve (normal adults, study IV)*

	Methylphenidate	
	0.15 mg/kg	0.30 mg/kg
N	5.00	10.00
GH	0.22	0.27
PRL	−0.32*	−0.47*
Mood	0.19	−0.49*
BP—systolic	0.09	−0.11
BP—diastolic	0.15	−0.15
Pulse	0.23	−0.05

* Significant correlation at $p = 0.05$ level.

In the 0.15 mg/kg group, the mean correlation between serum level and PRL is significant [$F(1,14) = 14.22$, $p < 0.05$] as is the correlation between systolic and diastolic blood pressures [$F(1,4) = 30.61$, $p = 0.01$].

The 0.3 mg/kg group showed significant correlations between serum level and PRL [$F(1,9) = 799.24$, $p < 0.00001$], serum level and mood [$F(1,6) = 8.925$, $p < 0.05$], and systolic and diastolic blood pressure [$F(1,8) = 165.18$, $p < 0.00001$]. The first two of these correlations are higher in this group than in the 0.15 group; $F(1,13) = 9.44$, $p < 0.01$, and $F(1,10) = 5.3$, $p < 0.05$, respectively.

COMPARISON OF MPD TIME PROFILES IN HAC AND ADULTS

Subjects, Method

For 7 male HAC and 7 male volunteers in studies 3 and 4, it was possible to compare MPD pharmacokinetic curves and neuroendocrine correlates at five time points: 0, 60, 120, 240, and 480 minutes post-drug, following a 0.3-mg/kg dose.

Analysis, Results

Blood samples were drawn for the following (common to children and adults) times post-drug: 0 hr, 1 hr, 2 hr, 4 hr, and 8 hr. Serum levels of MPD, GH and PRL were available for 7 children and 7 adults at these times. These data were subjected to orthogonal polynomial regression analysis with age as a nested factor and time (of measurement) as a crossed factor. Additionally, for GH and PRL, MPD was entered into the regression as a repeated prediction.

MPD

The only significant time effects are for the quadratic [$F(1,12) = 69.91$, $p < 0.0001$, $r^2 = 0.42$] and cubic [$F(1,12) = 40.79$, $p < 0.0001$, $r^2 = 0.24$] components of the curve. Although the main effect of age is not significant ($F < 1.0$), the age × time component is significant linearly, $F(1,12) = 6.43$, $p = 0.026$. This reflects the smaller amount of MPD in children at 8-hours post-drug (1.11) to adults (2.71). Although statistically significant, the effect is not markedly robust ($r^2 = 0.017$).

GH

The only significant effect is for the cubic component of time ($F(1,12) = 6.52$, $p = 0.025$), reflecting the triphasic shape of the curve. Serum levels of MPD across time are not significantly predictive of GH, $F(1,47) = 3.54$, $p > 0.05$, $r^2 = 0.05$.

PRL

Both the quadratic and cubic components of the time effect are significant, $F(1,12) = 13.00$, $p = 0.0036$, $r^2 = 0.20$; and $F(1,12) = 20.07$, $p = 0.0008$, $r^2 = 0.105$, respectively. Age interacts with the quadratic component of time, $F(1,12) = 5.95$, $p = 0.03$, $r^2 = 0.093$. This reflects the much sharper decline over the first 2 hours (post-drug) in adults, compared to children, as well as the failure of adults to recover to predrug levels. Serum levels of MPD do not predict PRL, $F(1,47) < 1.0$, $r^2 = 0.002$.

CLINICAL CORRELATES OF MPD SERUM LEVELS WITH REPEATED SAMPLING

Method

Four inpatient HAC who completed the acute effects study, and who were determined to be favorable responders to the drug on clinical grounds, were maintained on MPD and followed over a 3-week period. At regular intervals during this period, subjects returned to the clinic at 8 a.m., having fasted from midnight. The clinic nurse administered the child's usual dose of MPD, and an hour later a blood sample was drawn for MPD serum levels, GH and PRL. Then the child was tested on the CPT with a wristwatch actometer on the nondominant arm. The child then attended his usual classroom, where direct behavior observations were made by a research assistant using an interval time sampling technique (Wahler *et al.*, 1976). After class, the teacher completed the abbreviated CTRS. All measures were locked to the time of drug administration. Three children were tested on 8 separate days; one child was tested on 6 days.

Analysis

For each child, 11 dependent measures were available for analysis: GH and PRL, correct responses and commission errors on the CPT, actometer score, CTRS total score, mean CTRS scores for the hyperactivity and distractibility items, and direct observations of fidgeting, attentive and oppositional behavior in the classroom. Scores on each measure were correlated with the subject's 1-hour MPD serum level for that day.

Results

One-hour MPD serum levels were highly variable within subjects. In subject 1, serum levels ranged from 6.7 ng/ml to 15.5; subject 2, 7.9 to 23.1; subject 3, 9.3 to 21.7; and subject 4, 1.6 to 6.0.

TABLE 5.9 *Within-subject correlations of MPD serum levels in 4 HAC on successive days*

	S-1	S-2	S-3	S-4	Mean
Number of trials	8.00	6.00	8.00	8.00	
Day	0.22	0.63	0.03	−0.62	0.07
GH	0.65	0.58		0.05	0.46
PRL	0.20	−0.82*		0.49	−0.14
Actometer	0.35	−0.41	−0.35	−0.37	−0.21
CPTY		0.48	0.15		0.35
CPTN		−0.30	0.14		−0.09
CTRS—Total		−0.03	−0.76*	0.51	−0.16
CTRS—hyperactivity		−0.07		0.46	0.22
CTRS—distractibility		0.32	−0.12	0.29	0.17
ECOF	−0.15	−0.01	0.55	0.57	0.37
ECAT	0.15	0.16	−0.51	−0.59	−0.21
ECOP	−0.57	0.33	0.46		0.07

* $p < 0.05$; (1.85 significant correlations would be predicted by chance alone).
S = subject; Day = number of days from initiation of treatment; CPTY = continuous performance task, correct responses; CPTN = CPT, false alarms; ECOF = behavior observations, fidgetting; ECAT = behavior observations, attention; ECOP = behavior observations, oppositional behavior.

Despite this day-to-day variability, MPD serum levels were reliable. The mean correlation (for all subjects) between MPD serum levels on day N and day $N + 1$ was 0.89; thus, no less than 78% of the variance in serum levels on day $N + 1$ was attributable to the serum level on the earlier testing day.

There was no pattern of change in MPD serum levels relative to time; the mean correlation between serum levels and number of days since the subject first began taking the drug on a regular basis was $r = 0.07$ (NS).

There was no significant correlation, within subjects, between MPD serum levels and scores obtained on clinical measures of response. There are 33 correlation coefficients listed in Table 5.9; only 2 are significant at the $p = 0.05$ level. None of the mean correlations (Fisher's r to z transform) achieved significance.

DISCUSSION

MPD serum levels are reliable from a methodologic standpoint and from a statistical standpoint as well. However, MPD serum levels in a given individual are also quite variable, on a day to day basis, and this variability does not relate to the clinical variability which also occurs in HAC who take the medication on a daily basis. The pharmacokinetic profile of MPD is well-defined, and similar across studies of HAC and normal adults, although clearance of the drug is more rapid in children. Along the pharmacokinetic time profile of the drug, occasional associations can be demonstrated with certain measures, such as the neuroendocrine response and the euphoric response in adults. However, neither 1-hour serum levels nor any other pharmacokinetic parameter correlates with any of the host of measures employed to measure drug response in HAC. In the within-subjects analyses, occasional correlations may be found: the secretion of GH and PRL follows a pattern that reflects the pharmacokinetic profile of the drug. MPD serum levels, however, do not distinguish between drug responders and nonresponders; they are not correlated with the occurrence or severity of toxic effects; and they are not reflected, in the between-groups analyses, in correlated changes in any of the dependent measures.

Three reports in the literature suggest that MPD bloods levels may, in fact, be correlated with clinical response. They are, however, preliminary reports based on limited kinds of response measures in relatively small samples of children. Kupietz *et al.* (1982) reported a study of 5 HAC on chronic MPD treatment, who had full pharmacokinetic time profiles after their usual morning of MPD, while a learning task was administered along the course of the curve. The association between plasma concentrations of MPD and learning errors was tested by regression analysis. However, the regression did not, apparently, test the relative impact of time (along the curve) or dose on the variance in learning scores. A reanalysis of the data revealed no significant autocorrelations (within subjects) between MPD blood levels and learning errors.

Shaywitz *et al.* (1982) reported a study of 21 HAC on MPD at different doses. "Peak" MPD levels were said to be "significantly correlated to the percentage of improvement" on the CTRS ($r = 0.05$, $p < 0.02$ or $r = 0.771$, $p < 0.001$; two statistics are given for the same data). This contention is hard to understand, since the blood samples for MPD analysis were drawn at different times after drug administration in different children. In many cases the drug was actually administered by parents before the child came to the clinic.

In neither study was an attempt made to partial out the effects of dose on clinical response. The clinically essential question, after all, is not whether blood levels correlate with response, but whether any additional variance in response is attributable to blood levels after correction for variance in response attributable to dose. In other words, will blood levels predict any more about the patient's clinical response than dose will? In a third study (Winsberg *et al.*, 1980), this statistical manipulation was done, and, although blood levels were apparently associated with response, no additional variance in response was explained by blood levels after the effects of dose were partialled out.

On the basis of the research described herein, we conclude that MPD serum levels are not statistically related to clinical response, nor are they likely to prove clinically helpful. The reason for this dissociation may reside in the selective affinity of MPD for different tissues. For example, in preclinical studies conducted by colleagues in North Carolina, rat brain levels of MPD peaked earlier and at much higher concentrations than serum levels after intravenous or oral administration (Patrick *et al.*, 1984). Another possible explanation may be the lack of stereochemical specificity of the present MPD assay, which fails to distinguish between d- and l-enantiomers or threo-MPD. If the d- and l-isomers do, in fact, possess differential activity, then it is likely that the stereospecific assay would reveal significant correlations with clinical response. A third explanation may be pharmacodynamic rather than pharmacologic; that is, MPD response may be a function of neural sensitivity to the drug, rather than to drug level per se.

It is, therefore, concluded that MPD blood level determinations will probably not serve to improve the clinical management of HAC. To support this conclusion, it is worthwhile to translate the research findings presented above into actual clinical situations where one might hope that blood level determinations could make a difference in the clinical management of patients.

1. Patients who fail to respond to MPD may prove to have low blood levels; monitoring blood levels may turn apparent nonresponders into responders. This argument was actually advanced by Shaywitz *et al.* (1982), who described "three children judged to be nonresponders based upon observations of parents, physicians and school personnel." Two of the children were receiving 0.3 mg/kg and had 2-hour blood levels of 1 to 2 ng/ml; the third was receiving 0.6 mg/kg with a 2-hour level of 6.8 mg/ml. No further information about these children was given, however. For example, did higher doses or higher blood levels turn these patients into MPD responders? If so, did serum blood level determinations influence clinical decisions in a meaningful way, or could the dose simply have been titrated upwards? The authors maintain that "all three children who failed to respond had levels less than 7 ng/ml." This contention is based, however, on a clinical experiment with 26 children, only 21 of whom had systematic clinical response data. The data from our study of 55 ADD-H, in which clinical and laboratory evaluations were much more extensive, simply do not support this argument. In fact, serum levels above 7 ng/ml were found in substantial numbers of nonresponders; there was no significant difference between serum levels of responders and nonresponders. In the management of nonresponders, it is our experience that simple upward titration of the MPD dose is a satisfactory practice. Further, it is clear that intraindividual variation in MPD blood levels will limit the usefulness of a single blood level determination for clinical decisionmaking.

Finally, MPD blood levels are not significantly correlated with any of the response measures in the clinical studies described here. The variance in clinical response measures attributable to dose is not increased when knowledge of blood levels if introduced into the equation.

2. Toxic reactions may be prevented if blood levels are monitored carefully. If MPD blood levels could predict the development of toxic reactions, their usefulness to clinicians would be firmly established. In the acute effects study, however, no correlation between MPD blood levels and side effects was observed. Most of the acute side effects of MPD, moreover, such as anorexia, headache, insomnia and irritability, were readily apparent to parents and physicians. They are best treated by lowering the dose, irrespective of blood levels, by changing the schedule of drug administration, or by stopping the drug entirely.

Sprague and Sleator (1977) reported subtle cognitive changes in HAC on higher doses of MPD. It would be interesting to know if such effects were better predicted by dose or by blood level. It would also be interesting to know if deterioration on the matching to sample task employed in Sprague's laboratory bears any relation to actual learning or performance in the classroom. Although it is conceivable that MPD blood level would be related to subtle cognitive changes, for example in a matching-to-sample task, but not to other clinical or laboratory measures of response (including cognitive measures like the Continuous Performance Task or the Matching Familiar Figures Test), it is not very likely.

The development of late side effects like growth suppression or tics is a third instance where blood levels measures could be clinically useful. However, growth suppression appears to be a rare event at doses that are commonly prescribed (Kalachnick *et al.*, 1982). No one knows how frequently tics may develop in stimulant-treated children, but they are probably relatively infrequent, too. The likelihood of actually capturing a substantial number of growth-retarded or tic children in a longitudinal study of MPD blood levels is very small. Nor is it likely that serial blood levels measures would improve or alter currently recommended practice. All children on stimulants require periodic measurement of height and weight, and regular examinations for motor or phonic tics.

3. Monitoring BL may improve the management of children who develop tolerance to the therapeutic effects of MPD. Since longitudinal follow-up studies on children on stimulant drugs have not been widely reported, it is difficult to say how frequently tolerance develops to the therapeutic effects of MPD or other stimulant drugs. On the basis of our research (Gualtieri *et al.*, 1984) and that of others (Quinn and Rapoport, 1975), tolerance does not seem to be a common event in the long-term treatment of HAC. Further, in our longitudinal study of 17 HAC followed after 11 to 66 months on MPD, there was no apparent decline in MPD blood levels over time. If tolerance to stimulant drugs does develop in a given child, it may be pharmacologic or pharmacodynamic; the results of our follow-up study suggest that when it does occur, it is probably the latter. In either event, a physician faced with the development of tolerance

would probably simply raise the dose until therapeutic effects were once again achieved, or until toxic effects supervened. It is hard to say how blood level monitoring would improve this practice.

Assay of MPD blood levels is not likely to be clinically useful. It is possible that future studies will uncover a hitherto undiscovered link between some pharmacologic measures of MPD activity and some clinical measure of response, but it is not likely that such developments will have much impact on clinical practice.

REFERENCES

American Psychiatric Association, Task Force on Nomenclature and Statistics: Diagnostic and Statistical Manual of Mental Disorders, 3rd Ed. Washington, APA, 1978.

Breese G, Gualtieri T, Mailman R, Mueller R, Youngblood W, Vogel R, Wilson J: Developmental neuropsychopharmacology: preclinical and clinical studies of the hyperkinetic syndrome. In Rasken, Robinson and Levine (eds): Age and the Pharmacology of Psychoactive Drugs. New York, Elsevier 1981, pp 63–78.

Chan YM, Soldin SJ, Swanson JM, *et al.*: Gas chromatographic/mass spectroscopic analysis of methylphenidate (Ritalin) in serum. Clin Biochem J 1980; 13:266–272.

Chan YM, Swanson JM Soldin SS, Thiessen JJ, Macleod SM, Logan W: Methylphenidate hydrochloride given with or before breakfast: II. Effects of plasma concentrations of methylphenidate and ritalinic acid. Pediatrics 1983; 72:56–59.

Egeland J, Weinberg RA: The matching familiar figures test: a look at its psychometric credibility. Child Develop 1976; 47:483–491.

Gaito J: Equal and unequal n and equal and unequal intervals in trend analyses. Educ Psychol Meas 1973; 37:283–289.

Goyette CH, Conners CK, Ulrich RF: Normative data on revised Conners Parent and Teacher Ratings Scales. J Abnorm Child Psychol 1978; 6:221–236.

Grant DA: Analysis-of-variance tests in the analysis and comparison of curves. Psychol Bull 1956; 53:141–150.

Gualtieri CT, Wargin W, Kandy R, Shen C, Patrick K, Youngblood W, Mueller R, Breese G: Clinical studies of methylphenidate serum levels in children and adults. J Am Acad Child Psychiat 1982; 1982a; 21:19–26.

Gualtieri CT, Wargin W, Kandy R, Youngblood W, Breese GR: The effects of eating and fasting on the absorption of methylphenidate. Res Commun Psychiat Behav 1982b; 7:381–384.

Gualtieri CT, Hicks RE, Mayo JP, Schroeder SR, Lipton MA: The persistence of stimulant effects in chronically treated children: Further evidence of an inverse relationship between drug effects and placebo levels of response. Psychopharmacology 1984; 83:44–47.

Hungund BL, Perel JM, Hurwic MJ, Sverd J, Winsberg BG: Pharmacokinetics of methylphenidate in hyperkinetic children. Br J Clin Pharmacol 1979; 8:571–576.

Kalachnick JE, Sprague RL, Slcator EK, Cohen MN, Ullmann RK: Effect of methylphenidate hydrochloride on stature of hyperactive children. Dev Med Child Neurol 1982; 24:586–595.

Kupietz SS, Winsberg BG, Sverd J: Learning ability and methylphenidate plasma concentration in hyperkinetic children. J Am Assoc Child Psychiat 1982; 21:27–30.

Ostrom CW: Time series analysis: regression techniques. Beverly Hills, Sage Publications, 1978.

Patrick KS, Kilts, CD, Breese GR: Synthesis of deuterium-labelled methylphenidate, p-hydroxymethylphenidate, ritalinic acid and p-hydroxyritalinic acid. J Labelled Comp Radiopharm 1982; 9:485–490.

Patrick KS, Ellington KR, Breese GR: Distribution of methylphenidate and p-hydroxymethylphenidate in rat. J Pharmacol Exp Ther 1984; 231:61–65.

Patrick K, Ellington K, Breese G, Kilts C: Gas chromatographic mass fragmentographic analysis of methylphenidate and p-hydroxymethylphenidate using deuterated internal standards. J. Chromatography Biomedical Applications 1985, 343:329–338.

Quinn PO, Rapoport JL: One-year follow-up of hyperactive boys treated with imipramine or methylphendiate. Am J Psychiat 1975; 132:241–245.

Rosvold E, Mirsky R, Sarason I, Bransome E, Beck L: A continuous performance test of brain damage. J Couns Psychol 1956; 20:343–350.

Routh DK, Schroeder CS, O'Tuama L: Development of activity level in children. Dev Psychol 1974; 10:163–168.

Shaywitz SE, Hint RD, Jatlow P, Cohen DJ, Young JG, Pierce RN, Anderson GM, Shaywitz BA: Psychopharmacology of Attention Disorder: pharmacokinetic, neuroendocrine and behavioral measures following acute and chronic treatment with methylphenidate. Pediatrics 1982; 69:688–694.

Sprague RL, Sleator EK: Methylphenidate in hyperkinetic children: differences in dose effects on learning and social behavior. Science 1977; 198:1274–1276.

Sunshine I, Jatlow P: Methodology for analytical toxicology. In Sunshine I, Jatlow P (eds): Methodology for Analytical Toxicology. Vol II. Boca Raton, FL, CRC Press 1982.

Wahler RG, House AE, Stambaugh EE: Ecological Assessment of Child Problem Behavior. New York, Pergamon Press, 1976.

Wargin W, Patrick K, Kilts C, Gualtieri CT, Ellington K, Mueller RA, Kraemer C, Breese GR: Pharmacokinetics of methylphenidate in man, rat and monkey. J Pharmacol Exp Ther 1983; 226:382–386.

Weinsberg BG, Hungund BL, Perel JM: Pharmacological factors of methylphenidate metabolism in behaviorally disordered children. Psychopharmacol Bull 1980; 16:69–71.

Weinsberg BG, Kupietz SS, Sverd J, Hungund BL, Young NL: Methylphenidate oral dose plasma concentrations and behavioral response in children. Psychopharmacology 1982; 76:329–332.

6

Differential Psychopharmacology of Methylphenidate and the Neuro-psychology of Childhood Hyperactivity

ROBERT E. HICKS AND C. THOMAS GUALTIERI

EDITOR'S SYNOPSIS

The authors discuss the principal of rate dependency (RD) which Hicks had presented in the previous volume of this series. The strongest proposition relative to RD is that *the rate of responding completely determines the effect of a given dose of a drug*, other variables influencing the drug effect only indirectly by affecting rates of responding. Hicks presents an alternative hypothesis and has reviewed the whole topic in 1984. To clarify RD affect in hyperactivity, the authors performed a clinical experiment with 55 hyperactive children treated with MPH. Drug effects were analyzed and presented in alternate ways: (a) by employing classic RD methods, and (b) by employing analysis-of-variance with orthogonal polynomial regression.

The authors present an elegant mathematical analysis of RD functions for a large number of variables. However, they concluded that:

> It would appear that an RD analysis provides virtually no direct information concerning the direction or magnitude of the drug effect, nor of the relationship between responses on and off drug. In contrast, regression of (absolute values of) drug responses on placebo responses is an easy-to-grasp, mathematically justified technique for examining the homogeneity of drug effects and relationships between responses on and off drug.

Most of the measures change linearly with increasing dose and none of the quadratic components reached statistical significance. Thus, there appears to be no justification for a logarithmic (or any other kind) of transformation on these data that is not dictated by an explicit theory (Tukey, 1977).

The authors propose that: (a) a principal effect of stimulant drugs is to *canalize* various parameters of arousal and reactivity; (b) HAC (hyperactive children) are characterized by (i.e., possess the trait of) excessive variability, both in rate and magnitude of change, in arousal level and reactivity; (c) excessively inconsistent arousal and reactivity are frequently detrimental to attention, performance and social behavior; and (d) stimulant drugs thereby affect HAC more consistently across time, and with greater magnitude at any particular time, than they do control subject, as a consequence of their excessive variability. HAC are not "underaroused"; they are excessively variable in their level of arousal. Stimulants do not only increase low arousal levels but also lower high levels. Their effect is to canalize response to within more adaptive boundaries; a homeostatic effect (Gualtieri *et al.*, 1983).

The authors then discuss a neural substrate for ADDH. They discuss the similarities between childhood hyperactivity and frontal syndrome (FS). They propose that the mechanism responsible for these patients' failure in various conditional emotional paradigm may be limbic-frontal dissociation, that may be the core of symptomatology in both ADDH and FS. Lack of persistence on an extended action plan could be due to the frontal lobe's failure to influence the limbic system in generating motivation sufficient to sustain performance or failure of the limbic system to communicate motivational influences which are generated to frontal areas. This would also be consistent with the lack of foresight characteristic of both syndromes in the limbic evaluation of probable outcomes of various strategic alternatives, not available for frontal decision processes.

The authors conclude with the following summary:

> The contribution of behavioral pharmacology to the study of childhood hyperactivity is not to be found in the principle of rate-dependency, which we have shown is not relevant to the actual analysis of stimulant drug effects in a clinical study of HAC. Rather, the major contribution is to emphasize the importance of appreciating the state of the organism as an element which may influence the stimulant drug response. A consideration of this point of view leads to the hypothesis that HAC are characterized by the trait of widely varying states; the parameters of response are widely set, and oscillations are extreme and unpredictable within these parameters. Thus, the disorder is one of "dyshomeostatis," and the action of stimulant drugs serves as a homeostat. The neural basis for such a dysequilibratory disorder is postulated to lie in the frontal-striatal DA system and, in this context, the comparison between HAC and adult patients with the FS is salient and enlightening. Thus, the hyperkinetic syndrome is postulated to represent a genetically determined disorder or a dysmaturation of orbitofrontal DA systems.
>
> The frontal-striatal theory of childhood hyperactivity is heuristic. On the basis of this theory, it is hypothesized that HAC will exhibit dissociated deficits on neuropsychologic tasks, which measure frontal lobe dysfunction, and that stimulant drugs will selectively improve performance on these tasks.

Regretfully this chapter was replaced by the Editor's Synopsis for reasons of publication and since similar material may be found in: Evan

RW, Gualtieri CT, Hicks RE: A neuropathic substrate for standard drug effects in hyperactive children. *Clin. Neuropharm.*, 9:264–281, 1986 and other publications. Copies of the original chapter may be obtained from Robert E. Hicks, Ph.D., Department of Psychiatry, Wing B, 207H, University of North Carolina School of Medicine, Chapel Hill, North Carolina 27514.

REFERENCES

Gualtieri CT, Hicks RE, Mayo JP: Hyperactivity and homeostasis. J. Am. Acad. Child Psychiat., 22:382–384, 1983.

Hicks RE, Perez-Reyes M, Mayo JP, Gualtieri CT: Cannabis, atropine, and temporal information processing. Neuropsychobiology, 12:229–237, 1984.

Tukey JW: Exploratory Data Analysis. Reading, MA: Addison-Wesley, 1977.

7

Control System Instability in Hyperactive Children

MARCEL KINSBOURNE

Extensive investigation has failed to vindicate the catecholamine hypothesis as an explanation of hyperactive behavior (see Brown *et al.*, 1984 and discussion in volume II of this series). Resting catecholamine metabolite levels have not been shown conclusively to be abnormal; though stimulant drugs are known to control catecholamine metabolism, their therapeutic effects are not consistently related to changes in urine levels of catecholamine metabolites. Even serum levels of the drugs themselves relate only loosely to their therapeutic effects. It follows that alternative models for the mechanism of hyperactivity should be investigated.

Alternatives to the catecholamine deficiency model are the control system models; consequently we considered control system bias and instability as models of the hyperactive state.

Behavior dimensions (cognitive style or personality) are considered to be under the control of reciprocal balance between opponent processors. The momentary status of such a dimension is determined by the vector resultant of the opponents' relative excitation levels. Successful adaptation depends on the ability to shift this balance, and thus the direction of the vector, in flexible response to changing situational demands. Two patterns of malfunction in such a system can be envisaged: (a) *bias*, such that one of the two opposing processors dominates in most instances, rendering the individual inflexible on relevant behavioral dimensions; and (b) *instability*, underdampering, leading to fluctuating behavioral states for endogenous reasons, which are maladaptive because they are orthogonal to environmental demands. Whether a control system bias is reflected in abnormal neurotransmitter metabolite levels in body fluids depends on whether the opponent processor uses the same or different neurotransmitters. Given that no such imbalances have yet been discovered in hyperactivity, we will provisionally presume that the implicated control systems use a common neurotransmitter. We suggest, then, that for possibly diverse reasons (selective structural damage, underdevelopment, underactivation) system controlling variables, such as amount of reflectiveness or impact on behavior of the anticipation of negative consequences, are in imbalance in hyperactive children.

When an acute dose of relevant neurotransmitter is presented (directly or indirectly), the system in imbalance will swing toward the opposite state, overshooting if the system is unstable. The effective stimulus would be the rate of change in neurotransmitter level rather than the changed steady state level. Once the chemical impulse is delivered, the time course of the system's swing and ultimate return to its prior biased situation would depend on the properties of the system. Correspondingly, the behavioral effect of stimulant administration precedes any substantial rise in catecholamine levels in bodily fluids. Further, the time-response characteristic of the behavioral effect is the same for amphetamine and methylphenidate, although the chemical half-life of amphetamine in plasma is far longer. Further consistent is the finding that slow release d-amphetamine and methylphenidate have, if anything, a shorter duration of behavioral effect than the regular product, rather than the longer duration of action to be expected if, while in active form in the body, it was correcting some existing deficiency. The generally observed noncorrespondence between effective dose levels of stimulants and milligram per kilogram of body weight formulations further supports the notion that the stimulant drug jolts a skewed control system rather than corrects an existing deficiency.

If a phasic response to changing levels of catecholamine is a necessary condition for the effective control of hyperactive behavior by stimulant therapy, then several other phenomena fall into place. That tolerance to the stimulant does not occur would be explained by the fact that it clears the system once or twice daily. The inverted U-shaped curve of performance change with increasing dosage could, at least partly, be due to persisting effects of individual doses merging into each other, reducing the amplitude of change at each administration. In other words, as one increases the dose, the base-levels against which each subsequent dose takes effect is raised, reducing the possible range of further therapeutically effective changes in level of neurotransmitter. Of course, toxic effects at higher dose levels might blend with this proposed mechanism. It would follow that the much complained-of intermittency of currently employed stimulant regimens is precisely what permit them to be effective. Round-the-clock steady levels would, by this model, have no therapuetic effect at all.

If we assume that the drug-induced change in the level of neurotransmitter "perturbs" a biased control system to an extent proportional to dose level, then what follows is determined by the status of the balance between opponent processes. The more biased control system would be expected to be affected more powerfully, even to the point of overshooting the condition of equal balance. Systems already in equal balance would be little affected. Such a situation would yield functions of the type described by Hicks (1985) and colleagues and by ourselves (1985) in Volume 2 of this series. The amount of change from the placebo to the drug state would be proportionate to the extent to which the subject occupies an extreme position on the placebo. The correlation between placebo with drug minus placebo would also increase with successive increases in dosage. Both Hicks *et al.* and ourselves have found many instances of such relationships experimentally, and others can be derived from the literature by appropriate reanalysis of data there presented.

The control system model can account for a recurring finding, that no "deficiency" model can explain the fact that acute stimulant administration can have opposite effects, depending only on the base-state of the recipient. The "perturbation" model of stimulant effect explains why the same dosage will dampen activity in one individual, increase it in another; render one person more cautious, another more impulsive, and so forth. Hicks *et al.*'s treatment of the "rate dependency" principle has been invaluable in revealing its power and generality, and, as we have shown, assists in the formulation of new and potentially more viable models for the set of developmental personality disorders commonly known as hyperactivity.

Note: There was no discussion of Dr. Kinsbourne's stimulating paper because he was, unfortunately, unable to attend the symposium and mailed his paper. Eds.

REFERENCES

Brown GL, Ebert MH, Minichiello M: Biochemical and pharmacological aspects of attention deficit disorder. In Bloomingdale (ed.): Attention Deficit Disorder: Identification, Course and Rationale. New York, Spectrum Publications, 1985, pp 93–130.

Hicks RE, Gualtieri CT, Mayo JP, Schroeder SR, Lipton MA: Methylphenidate and homeostasis: drug effects on the cognitive performance of hyperactive children. In Bloomingdale (ed.): Attention Deficit Disorder: Identification, Course and Rationale. New York, Spectrum Publications, 1985, pp 131–141.

Kinsbourne M: Base-state dependency of stimulant effects on the cognitive performance of hyperactive children. In Bloomingdale (ed.): Attention Deficit Disorder: Identification, Course and Rationale. New York, Spectrum Publications, 1985, pp 143–154.

8

Measurement of Serum Concentrations and Behavioral Response in ADDH Children to Acute Doses of Methylphenidate

JAMES M. SWANSON

This chapter covers three topics: first, the use of laboratory measures of learning to document direction-of-response and dose-response characteristics of ADD patients to acute doses of stimulant drugs; second, the pharmacokinetics of methylphenidate (MPH) in ADDH children; third, how serum concentrations of MPH relate to cognitive response.

COGNITIVE RESPONSE TO STIMULANTS

Task specificity of response to stimulants must be recognized and considered when choosing laboratory tasks to measure response to stimulant medication. Weiss and Laties (1962) emphasized this point in their classic review of the effects of stimulant drugs on normal adults, as did we in a research program started in 1975 at the Hospital for Sick Children, in Toronto. Marcel Kinsbourne and I addressed this topic as it relates to classifying ADD children as favorable or adverse responders to stimulant medication (Swanson and Kinsbourne, 1976; Swanson *et al.*, 1978; Swanson and Kinsbourne, 1978; Swanson *et al.*, 1979; Swanson and Kinsbourne, 1979; Hiscock *et al.*, 1979; Kinsbourne and Swanson, 1980; Swanson and Kinsbourne, 1980; Swanson *et al.*, 1982). We have emphasized that assessments based on performances on a "low level intellectual task" (using the terminology of Weiss and Laties, 1962) may overestimate the favorable response to stimulant medication. In some ways, this is a variant of the Sprague and Sleator (1977) proposal suggesting different dose-response functions for different tasks. An assessment based on performance on low level task will result in a higher optimal dose (in Sprague's terminology) or identify more favorable responders (in our terminology) than performance on a high level task. We have suggested, as have Sprague and Sleator (1977), that a learning task may be an appropriate high level task for measuring response to stimulant medication in ADD children and that its use may protect a significant minority of ADD children (the adverse responders in our terminology) from mistreatment with stimulant drugs. In the general population of ADD children, its use may protect favorable responders from inappropriately high doses of stimulant drugs (in Sprague's terminology). In modern terminology, a high level task may be described as effortful (Hasher and Zacks, 1979) and a low level task may be one that requires minimal use of central processing capacity.

Our selection of the paired associate learning (PAL) task, as a high level or effortful task, was based on the literature of the 1960's and studies of effects of stimulants on normal adults (Weiss and Laties, 1962; Burns *et al.*, 1967, Smith, 1967) as well as on hyperactive children (Conners *et al.*, 1968). We have suggested before (Swanson and Kinsbourne, 1979) that performance on the PAL test produces a U-shaped dose-response curve and this paper suggests that this is a crucial factor in the choice of an effortful or high level task. Other high level or effortful tasks have been recommended on the same grounds. Based on the shape of the dose-response curve, for example, the data of Sprague and Sleator (1977) may be interpreted to suggest that in their scanning task, the 9- and the 15-item display conditions (but not the 4-item display condition) are effortful or high level tasks because performance on them produces U-shaped dose-response curves, while the 4-item display condition does not.

A short review on the methodology of our version of the PAL test is appropriate at this point. Initially, we (Swanson and Kinsbourne, 1976), used naturalistic pictures of animals, paired with names of 4 Canadian cities. A new set of pictures was used for each test to establish an "A-B, C-B" paradigm with minimal practice effects (Kausler, 1974). The total number of errors a child made before reaching a criterion of "two perfect recitations of the list" was the measure of performance. About 20 to 30 minutes per test were required to reach this criterion of performance. Our basic research strategy was to establish a stable level of performance for new learning and then see if the child's performance level (number of errors) changes when medication is given under double-blind conditions. In several studies, we (Swanson and Kinsbourne, 1976; Dalby *et al.*, 1977; Swanson *et al.*, 1978) used the PAL test to evaluate the acute response to medication under double-blind conditions within a single day. In this one-day paradigm, capsules were administered in the morning (9:00 a.m.) and in the afternoon (12.00 p.m.). Only one of the capsules would contain medication, and would be given either in the morning capsule and placebo in the afternoon capsule, or vice versa. Acute changes in performance on the PAL test were observed to be associated with the administration of MPH in this double-blind protocol, but not all of the observed changes were favorable. Based on several studies, we defined a 25% drug-related decreased in errors (relative to placebo performance) on the PAL test as a reflection of a favorable cognitive response, and a 10% drug-related increase in errors as a reflection of an adverse cognitive response. Between these boundaries, a classification as a nonresponder would be appropriate. Theoretically, by increasing the dose and retesting, a nonresponder would be pushed toward one of these cutoff boundaries. (In practice, we usually consider adverse responders and nonresponders together as a group to contrast with the favorable responder group). The dose of MPH was $5 \rightarrow 20$ mg per administration.

In our research, other tests that do not require new learning, such as a continuous performance task (Swanson *et al.*, 1979), one trial incident recall task (Thurston *et al.*, 1979), a dichotic listening task (Hiscock *et al.*, 1979), or working arithmetic problems (Pelham *et al.*, 1980), did not produce U-shaped dose-response curves or do not identify as many adverse responders as does the PAL test. The Sprague and Sleator (1977) task may be an exception, since it is more a scanning task than a learning task in the classic sense.

As discussed elsewhere, this use of the PAL test is merely one way to quantify the "diagnostic drug trial" procedure proposed long ago by Laufer and Denhoff (1957). According to their recommendations, a provisional diagnosis of ADD (or as they called it, the hyperkinetic-impulse disorder) should be made, based on observations and/or reports of behavior. Next, this provisional diagnosis should be evaluated by a trial on stimulant medication. The provisional diagnosis is confirmed by a favorable response, or refuted by an adverse response. Laufer and Denhoff (1957) did not specify how to measure response but we have suggested that the PAL test be used to quantify the cognitive response to stimulant medication. Along with the double-blind paradigm, this provides an objective and systematic way of carrying out Laufer and Denhoff's (1957) diagnostic drug trial. Over the past several years, we have found that the PAL test, when used in the medication assessment procedures described above on clinic referred cases of ADD, confirmed the provisional diagnosis in about 60% of the cases by a favorable cognitive response, and refuted it in about 40% of the cases by an adverse response (Swanson and Kinsbourne, 1977).

The validity of the diagnostic drug trial has been questioned (Rapoport *et al.*, 1978; Taylor, 1983). We have discussed this issue elsewhere (Swanson and Kinsbourne, 1978, 1979, 1980) but, in my opinion, this issue has not yet been resolved. However, the Laufer and Denhoff (1957) procedure is still used by most clinicians when they start a new patient on stimulants, or when they titrate medication levels. For example, Goodman and Gillman (1980) recommended a titration procedure for increasing daily dose up to 2 mg/kg or until side effects occur and Barkley (1981) recommends a more systematic but similar procedure with titration based on parent and teacher reports via questionnaires. Use of a double-blind procedure may remove an obvious bias from the usual clinical procedures (Varley and Turpin, 1984) but reliance on questionnaires or ratings does not provide a measure of high level or effortful cognitive activity directly in the child. The use of a learning task or an effortful task may add an important dimension to the standard subjective evaluations derived from parents and teacher reports (Sprague and Sleator, 1977; Swanson and Kinsbourne, 1978). It is important to note that the addition of both the double-blind protocol and the use of an effortful task to the usual clinical procedures should operate to decrease the number of patients classified as favorable responders to medication. Using a double-blind procedure with cognitive tests, more subtle forms of the adverse response patterns should be detected than in the traditional clinical titration method, due to the sensitivity of the high level or effortful test for measuring cognitive toxicity (Sprague and Sleator, 1977).

The literature (e.g., Weiss and Laties, 1962; Sprague and Sleator, 1977; Swanson and Kinsbourne, 1978) clearly indicates that any evaluation of response to medication is highly dependent on the type of task used to measure that response. The Sprague and Sleator (1977) visual scanning task, or the memory scanning task used by Pelham (1986) and Sergeant (1986) may be as sensitive as the PAL test for measuring cognitive toxicity or adverse response to medication but I know of no other test that would identify a larger percentage of ADD children as adverse responders than the PAL task. In that way, the PAL test is a conservative test for assessing response to medication or for determining the optimal dose of medication.

USE OF THE PAL TEST

Two ways in which the PAL test has been used are: (a) as an aid to quantify the length of action of stimulant medication and (b) as a criterion variable for documenting overdose effects of stimulant medication.

In the mid 1970's, there were no studies on the serum half-life of MPD, despite the fact that it was one of the most widely used drugs in children. Presumably, this deplorable situation existed because the drug was approved for use before the present-day FDA requirements were established and enforced. In addition, in the early 1970's it was very difficult to measure serum concentrations of MPD (Bartlett and Egger, 1972; Faraj, 1974). In our early work, since serum concentrations of the drug were not available to estimate half-life in the usual way, we calculated behavioral half-life. This was done by testing subjects repeatedly throughout the day, after an acute dose of medication to generate time-response curves. Then, by inspecting group time-response curves, the peak level of performance could be identified and the time required for a 50% change as the drug effects dissipated determined as a measure of behavior half-life. We estimated that the behavioral half-life of MPD, based on the PAL test performance, was approximately 3 to 4 hours (Swanson *et al.*, 1978).

Most of our ADD patients classified as favorable responders show improved performance on the PAL test at doses of 5 to 10 mg of MPD. However, as we (Swanson *et al.*, 1978) observed when these favorable responders were given a higher dose of medication, an adverse or overdose response pattern can be elicited. These data reinforce the point made by Sprague and Sleator (1977) about task specificity and dose response. We (Swanson *et al.*, 1978) observed a nonmonotonic dose-response curve for performance on the PAL test as a function of the dose of MPD, as Sprague and Sleator (1977) did for their scanning task in the 9 and 15 items display conditions. (In an analysis of variance, the statistical evidence for this can be derived from a significant quadratic effect in an orthogonal polynomial decomposition of the main effect of dose). One should not expect this type of cognitive toxicity to emerge for ratings of behavior (Sprague and Sleator, 1977), nor for many simple laboratory tests (Swanson *et al.*, 1979; Thurston *et al.*, 1979; Hiscock *et al.*, 1979).

William Pelham and I (Pelham *et al.*, 1980) have used the PAL test to describe the dose-response functions for pemoline (PEM), another stimulant medication. In this study, 28 ADD children were given four doses of pemoline (18.75, 37.5, 75, and 112.5 mg) or placebo. Each dose was administered once a day (in the morning) for an entire week. Once a week, the children came to the laboratory (in groups of five or six) and were observed and tested for the entire day (8:30 a.m. to 4:30 p.m.). In addition to the PAL test, which requires new learning, an academic task requiring execution of a previously learned skill (working arithmetic problems) was given four times over the day (at 9:00 a.m., 11:00 a.m., 1:00 p.m. and 3:00 p.m.). The children were observed doing academic work in a model school room in the morning and afternoon. The Conners 10-item rating scale was used to assess behavior in this setting.

In this study, teacher ratings of behavior were best (lowest) and arithmetic performance was best (most problems worked) for the highest dose of mg pemoline PEM (112.5 mg). However, the optimal dose of PEM for effects on the PAL test was an intermediate dose level (75 mg). These data replicate and extend Sprague and Sleator's (1977) finding for MPD, suggesting that the optimal dose of stimulant medication for effects on learning was lower than that for effects on behavior. The data also demonstrate the ability of the PAL test to document overdose effects: the dose response function for the PAL test was nonlinear (a significant quadratic effect emerged in the decomposition of the main effect of dose in the ANOVA), in contrast to the linear dose-response function for teacher ratings of behavioral and for arithmetic performance.

The ability of a test to show overdose effects, even in favorable responders, fulfills a crucial criterion for the selection of a test for assessing response to stimulant medication. The test has demonstrated this property, in the Swanson *et al.*, (1978) study (for MPH) and in the Pelham *et al.* (1980) study (for PEM).

SERUM CONCENTRATIONS OF STIMULANT DRUGS

The therapeutic effects of some drugs are predicted better by serum concentration than by oral dose of drug. This may be due to individual differences in the absorption and/or metabolism of the drug. It seems reasonable to speculate, then, that this may explain individual variations in the clinically effective dose of MPH or PEM. In any group of hyperactive children receiving stimulant drugs, the oral dose required for a clinically significant response varies considerably across individuals (Schain and Reynard, 1975). Doses of MPH from 5 to 20 mg are recommended. The typical frequency of administration varies from once-a-day to three-times-a-day, resulting in a total daily dose of 5 to 60 mg. Doses of PEM from 18.75 to 112.5 mg are recommended and, even though once-a-day dosing is generally recommended, more frequent dosing may be necessary, especially in young children (Collier *et al.*, 1985).

Before 1980, little work was done relating serum concentration of stimulant drugs to their behavioral effect. In part, this was because of difficulties in the measurement of the most frequently used stimulant, MPH (Bartlett and Egger, 1972; Faraj *et al.*, 1974). However, several laboratories have solved the early problems and now have reported a serum level of MPH (Gualtieri *et al.*, 1982; Kupietz *et al.*, 1982; Shaywitz *et al.*, 1982). Recently, we (Soldin *et al.*, 1979; Chan *et al.*, 1980; Chan *et al.*, 1982; Tompkins *et al.*, 1982; Collier *et al.*, 1985) have studied the pharmacokinetics of MPH and PEM and related serum concentration of these drugs to behavioral effects.

We (Swanson and Soldin, in preparation) investigated the pharmacokinetics of MPH in ADD children who had been receiving the drug on a long-term basis. For our initial work, we selected patients taking the following oral doses (per administration) of MPH: 10 mg, 15 mg, 25 mg, 40 mg, 50 mg, 70 mg, and 100 mg. Some subjects who were taking extremely high doses of medication were included, even though we do not agree with this practice. The patient receiving 100 mg of MPD per administration was taking that amount four to six times per day. This is the largest dose of MPH we have encountered for the treatment of hyperactivity and assume that this patient had developed a tolerance to the drug. One of the questions we addressed in this extreme case was whether this was metabolic tolerance (in which the absorption and disposition of the drug was altered) or functional tolerance.

Patients were admitted to the Clinical Investigations Unit (CIU) of the Hospital for Sick Children in Toronto on the day before the investigation started. At that time their regular medication was stopped. At 7:30 a.m. on the next day patients were given a single oral dose of MPH equal to their usual morning dose. This amount varied from 10 to 100 mg across patients. Following the 7:30 a.m. dose, blood samples were taken from an indwelling catheter at 8:00 a.m., 9:30 a.m., 11:00 a.m. 12:00 noon, 1:30 p.m. 3:00 p.m. and 4:00 p.m. Breakfast was served at 8:30 a.m. and lunch at 12:30 p.m.

Initially, we used the high pressure liquid chromatographic (HPLC) analysis described by Soldin *et al.*, (1979a, 1979b) to measure serum drug (MPH) concentrations and its major metabolite, ritalinic acid (RA). We have established that a high correlation ($r = 0.84$) exists between levels of MPH and RA.

Serum levels and pharmacokinetics of MPH and RA are presented in Chan *et al.*(1983). Consider the serum levels of MPH and RA for the 2 patients who received the highest (100 mg) and the lowest (10 mg) doses in the Swanson *et al.* (in preparation) study. (As mentioned earlier, these doses had been established as clinically effective doses not by us but by others, as a result of long-term treatment and titration based on clinical criteria which did not include laboratory tests of learning). The patient receiving high doses of MPH showed correspondingly high serum concentrations of the drug and its metabolite. The peak serum concentration of RA was over 2000 μg/liter in the patient who took the 100-mg dose, compared to less than 200 μg/liter in the patient who took the 10 mg dose. Serum levels of MPH are lower than those of RA, but a similar dose relationship held: the peak serum level of MPH was over 170 μg/liter in the patient who received the 100 mg dose, while it was 40 μg/liter in the patient who received the 10 mg dose. This relationship held for six other patients, who were given from 10 to 70 mg of MPH. Overall, there was no evidence of impaired absorption or metabolism of MPH in children taking high doses of the drug.

A second purpose of this research was to compare serum half-life for the parent drug (MPH) and its metabolite (RA) across individuals. In several subjects, values for half-life were obtained both for MPH and RA (see Chan *et al.*, 1983). In some early reports (Bartlett and Egger, 1972; Faraj *et al.*, 1974) MPH levels were very low or undetectable shortly after the oral administration of 20 mg of the drug. But, in line with Milberg *et al.* (1975), we observed levels of MPH which, although lower than RA levels, were still detectable several hours after the administration of a low (10 or 15 mg) oral dose. In this series of studies (Swanson and Soldin, in preparation) the serum concentration of MPH and RA were highly correlated over time ($r > 0.84$), indicating that the pharmacokinetic information from MPH and RA serum levels is redundant. Thus, either the serum concentration of the drug (MPH) or its metabolite (RA) could be used to contrast half-life values across individuals, despite uncertainty about which substance mediates the central nervous system effect (Gal *et al.*, 1977). With HPLC procedures, the measurement of RA is easier than that of MPH, which requires gas chromatographic mass spectrometric (GC/MS) procedures for adequate sensitivity (Chan *et al.*, 1980). For this practical reason, we focused on the pharmacokinetics of RA in our initial study. In later studies, we measured both MPH and RA (Chan *et al.*, 1983) and found the half-life of the parent drug (MPH) in serum (2.1 hr) was shorter than that of its metabolite RA (3.4 hr).

The average half-life based on serum levels of RA was 3.37 ± 0.507 hr for the seven hyperactive children investigated in the present study. The half-life values did not differ much across individuals, or as a function of dose. The average half-life for the two patients who had clearly developed tolerance to MPH was 3.5 hours (for the 100-mg dose it was 4.2 hr, and for the 70-mg dose it was 2.8 hr), while the average half-life for the two patients taking ordinary doses was 3.17 hours (3.13 for the 10-mg dose and 3.21 for the 15-mg dose).

While values of half-life do not differ much across individuals in this sample of hyperactive children, they are substantially less than values previously reported in nonhyperactive adults (Faraj *et al.*, 1974). It remains to be determined whether this difference is due to a difference in the age of the patients (children versus adults), temperament (hyperactive versus normal), or to some other factor.

Previously, Swanson *et al.* (1978) estimated the behavioral half-life of MPH in hyperactive children, based on the time-response characteristics of their cognitive response to a single oral dose of the drug. That estimate (4.0 hr) is about the same as the value estimated here from serum levels of the metabolite RA (3.4 hr). Thus, the half-life of RA corresponds to the experimental estimates of the length of action of MPH.

An interesting difference in the correlation between serum concentration and behavioral effect seems to exist for the two primary stimulant medications, MPH and dextroamphetamine (d-amphetamine). We (Chan *et al.*, 1980, 1983) and others (Gualtieri *et al.*, 1982; Shaywitz *et al.*, 1982) have reported that peak serum concentrations of MPH coincide in time with peak behavioral and cognitive effects: both are manifested at about 2 hours after an acute administration of MPH. (Kupietz *et al.*, 1982, used a different method to obtain serum concentrations of MPH, and found a later peak time in a few subjects). On the other hand, the peak behavioral effect of d-amphetamine seems to occur before the peak serum concentration, which occurs at about 4 hours after its acute administration. This led Brown *et al.* (1979, 1980) to suggest that (a) the behavioral effects of d-amphetamine are greatest during the absorption phase (1 to 4 hours after an acute administration); (b) the behavioral effects are minimal after peak serum concentration is attained (4 hours after administration); (c) the half-life estimate (6.8 hours) observed during the elimination phase is not characteristic of the length and action of the behavioral effect. Thus, specific behavior and motor activity responses are not correlated with specific levels of d-amphetamine. In contrast, behavior effects seem to correlate directly with serum concentrations of MPH (Gualtieri *et al.*, 1982). The reasons for this basic difference are not clear.

Even though serum concentrations and behavioral effect are correlated for MPH, the clinical utility of serum concentrations is very limited. The absorption and disposition of MPH seems to be similar in those ADD children taking the usual doses (10 or 20 mg per administration) and those taking unusually high doses (70 to 100 mg). Half-life values are about the same for children taking these different doses. Peak serum concentrations vary directly with dose, so children who take high doses also have high serum levels of MPH. Thus, even though serum concentrations vary directly with dose and are highly correlated with behavioral effects across the day, there seems to be little use for the measure of serum concentration in practice, since it offers no information in addition to that derived from the oral dose of medication administered and knowledge of the time course effects.

SERUM CONCENTRATION AND BEHAVIORAL RESPONSE

Our next study of serum concentration of MPH addressed the issue of behavior response to different doses, to follow the pharmacokinetic investigation described above. We (Swanson and Soldin, in preparation) investigated dose-response patterns of several groups of hyperactive children: (a) those who had shown a long-term favorable response to a dose within the recommended range of 10 to 40 mg daily; and (b) those who required over 60 mg daily for a favorable response. The cognitive response was monitored by giving the PAL test at various times across the day, and blood samples were taken at the same times to monitor serum drug concentrations. Our purpose was to correlate behavior effects with serum concentration, with an emphasis on the cognitive effect of different doses of medication, as suggested by Sprague and Sleator (1977).

The doses of MPH in our patients had been determined by titration, by the child's regular pediatrician and we took them to be the established or historical dose of medication, not necessarily the optimal doses. The nature of the special group of ADD children receiving high doses of MPH must again be emphasized. These children started off on low doses of MPH but, over the years and in the eyes of their physician, the clinically significant effect of these drug doses had dissipated. The child's physician then recommended an increase in dose, a standard clinical practice. However, most patients do not develop a marked tolerance to MPH and this upward titration usually occurs perhaps once or twice at the most, resulting in moderate doses between 10 to 20 mg per administration. However, for the children in our high dose group, the process was repeated several times and high doses (up to 100 mg three times daily) resulted. Even though we do not agree with the use of such high doses, we did find this group of patients to be of considerable interest and thus selected them for investigation.

Patients entered the hospital on Sunday evening. Starting on Monday morning, blood samples were taken at the following times: 7:00 a.m., 8:00 a.m., 9:30 a.m., 11:00 a.m., 12:00 noon, 1:30 p.m., 3:00 p.m. and 4:00 p.m. Medication was administered three times a day: at 7:30 a.m., 11:30 a.m. and 3:30 p.m., to approximate usual clinical practice. The first day was a practice day. On the next 3 days, patients either received placebo, a low, or a high dose of MPH on a thrice daily basis. The order of these three conditions was counterbalanced across subjects. Since medication was given three times per day, we expected a steady state across the day so that a stable measurement of behavior effect and serum concentration could be obtained for each dose.

The dose for each patient was selected to be relevant to clinical as well as research questions. In the case of patients taking the usual or low doses, the questions were: "Has the optimal dose of medication been reached?" or, "Will a higher dose produce a better response?" These patients were tested on their established doses and on twice their established doses. In the case of patients taking a high dose an additional question was asked: "Has the optimal dose of medication been exceeded?" or, "Will a lower dose produce a better response?" These subjects were tested on their established doses, 50% of their established doses, and at 150% of their established doses.

After each blood sample was taken, the patients performed the PAL test (Swanson *et al.*, 1978) to allow us to monitor the cognitive effect of the drug. The 7:00 a.m. test was designed to wake the patient up, and the remaining seven tests were arranged to occur 30 minutes, 2 hours, or $3\frac{1}{2}$ hours after each dose of medication. We used the average performance over the seven tests in the placebo condition as a baseline. We expressed all scores as a percentage of this baseline score.

The data from the low-dose group, shown in Figure 8.1, indicate that fewer errors were made when patients received their established dose of medication (10 mg of MPH) than when they received placebo. This confirms that these patients were favorable responders to MPH at this dose. When their dose of medication was increased to 20 mg (exceeding their established dose), performance on the PAL test deteriorated. As

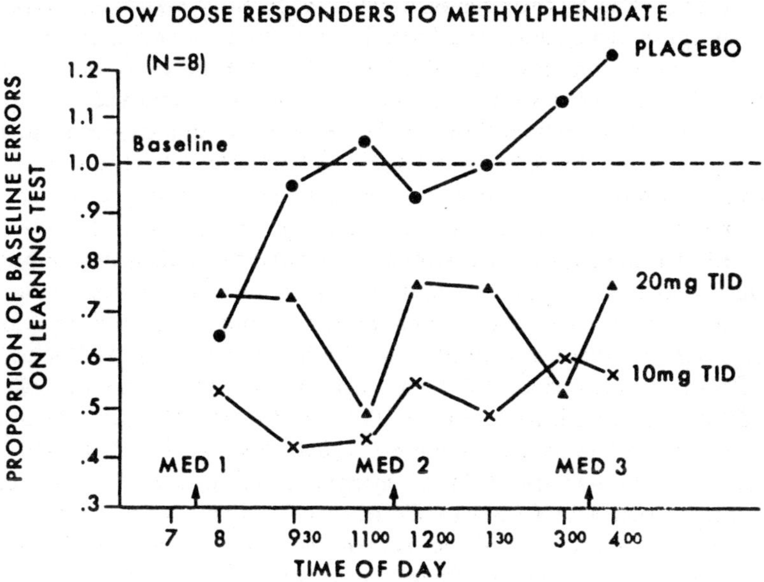

FIG. 8.1 Effect of Ritalin on learning.

shown in Figure 8.1, more errors were made on PAL tests on the day the high dose was administered than when the low dose was given. A trend analysis of the significant dose effect revealed a significant quadratic effect [$F(1,7) = 10.8$, $p < 0.002$], providing statistical support for the existence of an overdose effect on cognitive performance. The overdose response was most pronounced for the PAL test given 2 hours after the capsules were administered.

Thus, the results of our PAL test for the low-dose group (Swanson and Soldin, in preparation) indicated that the 10 mg, thrice daily dose was optimal for these patients and that the 20 mg thrice daily dose was excessive. The value of the serum concentration associated with the optimal response and the value of the toxic serum concentration associated with the overdose response should define the therapeutic range of serum concentrations for this group of patients. The average serum concentration of RA (the MPH metabolite) for the optimal dose of 10 mg three times a day varied across the day between 100 μg/liter and 200 μg/liter. The serum concentration of RA associated with the overdose response to 20 mg three times daily varied over the day between 250 μg/liter and 400 μg/liter. These data can be used to estimate the therapeutic range of serum concentration for RA (the MPH metabolite) for this group of ADD patients who respond favorably to the usual (10 mg) doses. The optimal range is between 100 and 200 μg/liter while over 250 μg/liter is the lower limit of the behaviorally toxic range (Swanson and Soldin, in preparation).

This study (Swanson and Soldin, in preparation) shows several interesting things. First, even with three-times-a-day dosing, there is a wide (twofold) variation in RA serum concentration across the day. If behavioral effect is related to serum concentration, then a corresponding variation in behavior should be expected. Second, the rapid decline in serum concentration is apparent for both the 10 and 20 mg doses, both after the first (7:30 a.m.) and after the second (11:30 a.m.) administration of the capsule that contained medication.

There are several critical questions concerning the group of patients who had developed tolerance and required high doses of methylphenidate in order to maintain a favorable clinical response. Whether the serum concentration (100 to 200 μg/liter) associated with the optimal behavioral response of these patients was the same as in the group of low-dose responders, despite the different oral dose requirements, was investigated. The data from the tolerant group are shown in Figure 8.2. First, it was necessary to establish the optimal behavior response in the group taking high doses. The data from the PAL test for the high dose group are presented in Figure 12.2. These patients were given three doses, in addition to the placebo treatment: (a) their established dose (average 45 mg); (b) 50% of their established dose (22.5 mg); and (c) 150% of their established dose (67.5 mg three times daily). The lower (50%) dose was

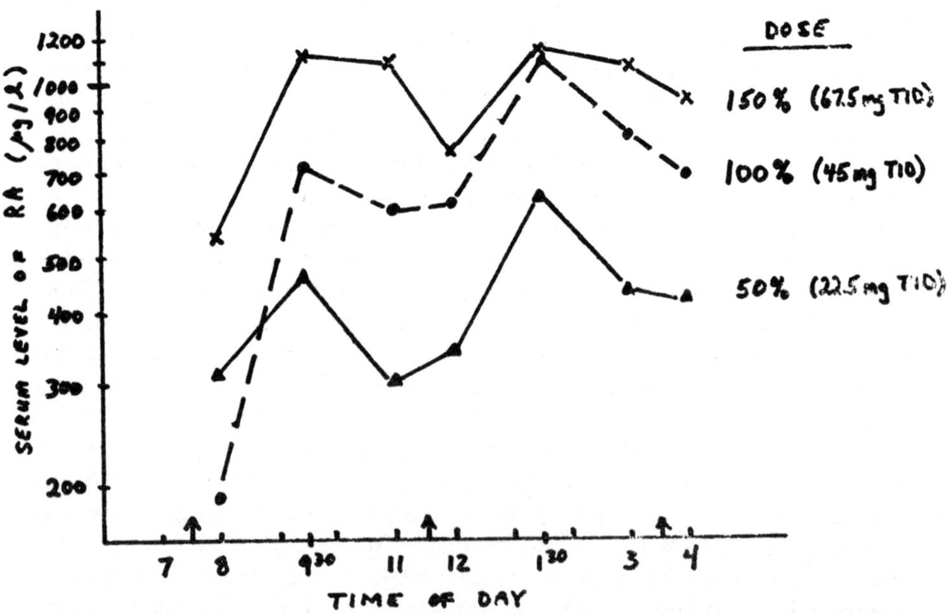

FIG. 8.2 Serum level of Ritalinic acid high dose group—$N = 5$.

given to determine whether a decrease in the historic dose would produce an improved cognitive response. We suspected that these patients might be overdosed on their established doses, which were very high (45 mg three times a day). The higher (150% dose was given to investigate whether the established dose was truly optimal, or if a higher dose would produce a better response or an overdose effect.

As shown in Figure 8.2, the average historic dose of 45 mg produced fewer errors than the placebo treatment, confirming that the patients responded favorably to such a high dose. This was somewhat surprising because we had hypothesized that these patients may have been inappropriately treated with these high doses (perhaps due to reliance on the behavior rather than cognitive effects to evaluate response and titrate dose).

Furthermore, when the dose was reduced by 50% (to 22.5 mg three times a day, which is still a high dose), cognitive performance of the patients in this group deteriorated relative to performance elicited by the higher dose, confirming the favorable response pattern. Also, extremely high doses failed to overdose these patients: even at the 150% (67.5 mg) dose, performance deterioration was not noted. Statistical support for this was obtained from a trend analysis of the learning data for this group; the linear component of the dose effect was significant, but the quadratic effect was not [$F(1,4) = 1.52$, $p < 0.25$].

We investigated whether the serum concentration of RA in those patients taking high doses differed from those taking low doses, we expected to find that these tolerant patients have low serum concentrations (e.g., in the 100 μg/liter to 200 μg/liter range) despite their high historic doses. If this were the case, then such high doses (average = 45 mg three times daily) for these patients would be understandable and decrease legitimate concerns about an apparently excessive amount of medication being used with this special group of tolerant patients.

However, this simplifying outcome did not occur (Swanson and Soldin, in preparation). This group of patients had serum concentration of RA ranging from 700 μg/liter to 1500 μg/liter (with their average established dose of 45 mg three times daily), compared to the optimal serum level of 100 μg/liter to 200 μg/liter for the nontolerant group (with their average established dose of 10 mg three times daily). Even when the dose was reduced by 50% to 22.5 mg three times a day, and performance on the learning test deteriorated, the serum concentrations of RA were still over three times higher (between 300 μg/liter and 600 μg/liter than those associated with the optimal response in the low (or standard) dose group. Wide variation across the day and the rapid decline in serum concentration after each administration in the three times-a-day dosing schedule were apparent in this tolerant group of ADD patients, just as in the group of ADD patients taking the usual (drug) dose of medication.

Why do some hyperactive children require a higher-than-usual dose of MPH to maintain a favorable response? Apparently the answer to this question will not be found by analyzing serum concentrations of the drug. Our data indicate that children who seem to require a high oral dose of MPH also have correspondingly high serum concentrations of the drug and its metabolite. The serum concentrations of MPH are directly related to oral dose, even in the unusual subgroup of ADD children who developed tolerance to the drug. Thus, the usefulness of serum concentration of the drug is very limited. Reliance on oral dose provides the same information obtained from serum concentrations.

SUMMARY

This research failed to demonstrate the clinical usefulness of serum concentration of MPH. A byproduct, however, is the extremely important information about behavioral response this research provided. The revised procedure for monitoring behavioral effects across the day represents a major improvement over the "one-day" paradigm in which performance at one point in time is observed. Since we gave the PAL test across the entire day when no medication (placebo) was given, we were able to make "time-of-day" adjustments, which were not possible in our previous one-day paradigm. The mean number of errors across the day in the placebo condition was subtracted from each score. That difference was then divided by the mean placebo score to yield a percentage (of the mean) score. Expressed in this way, the time-response curve on the placebo day reflects "time-of-day" effects. As shown in Figure 8.1, performance deteriorated across the day in the placebo condition in the presence of multiple testing and blood sampling. The performance was the best (fewest errors) on the first test, and worst at the end of the day.

Time-course effects in the three-times-a-day schedule (with a 4-hour dosing interval) extended the pattern established using the "one-day" paradigm (Swanson *et al.*, 1978). In the low-dose group, the maximal effect on learning occurred at about 2 hours after each administration. As shown in Figure 8.1, this was at 9:30 a.m. following the 7:30 a.m. capsule, and at 1:30 p.m. following the 11:30 a.m. capsule. The effect rapidly dissipated: by 11:00 a.m. following the 7:30 a.m. capsule, or by 3:00 p.m. following the 11:30 a.m. capsule, performance on the PAL test had deteriorated. (In the high dose condition, performance was impaired relative to the low dose condition but was still better than in the placebo condition. Even then, the rapid time course effects were apparent after each administration of a capsule. However, in this case the maximal effect 2 hours post administration reflected impairment, more errors, that dissipated over the next 2 hours).

CONCLUSIONS

In the low-dose group, the previously reported (Swanson *et al.*, 1978) favorable and overdose effects were documented, again using the PAL test. This confirms that these effects are not due to "regression to the mean" or chance, since multiple tests were given in each condition. This study, with the appropriate controls of multiple tests across an entire day in each drug condition, provided the best demonstration of the ability of the PAL test to reflect the cognitive effects of MPD. The overdose effect, or the U-shaped dose-response function, is particularly noteworthy. Of course, as Sprague and Sleator (1977) have pointed out, a dose-response analysis using other measures of response may not show overdose effects. The PAL task (or some other learning or effortful task) may provide additional data to the clinician for consideration but it is important to realize that this type of cognitive measure is likely to conflict with dose-response information from teachers and parent ratings (Sprague and Sleator, 1977) or from low level laboratory tasks.

GENERAL DISCUSSION

Dr. Thivierge: This kind of medication doesn't improve the long-term outcome on school performance. What was the rationale for giving these children such huge doses?

Dr. Swanson: The children were sent to me for evaluation. Half of those getting the medication have cognitive impairment associated with it even though teachers and parents think they are getting better. Medication is used because of the subjective ratings of parents or teachers. If you look at the curves I published in *Pediatrics* (Swanson *et al.*, 1978) only 5 of the 11 children who had been on medication for over 2 years were favorable responders. The others were adverse responders on cognitive tests, even though parent ratings showed all had improved. There is no long-term benefit from medication and one reason may be that many of the children who are getting medication are actually adverse responders cognitively, regrettably disregarded by clinicians, who ignored the work of Sprague and Sleator (1977) and of Sergeant (Chapter 1, this Volume).

Dr. Pelham: Why do you say those children are tolerant to medication as opposed to there being something different about their nervous system?

Dr. Swanson: At a starting dose of 10 mg three times daily they had good responses. Whenever the response disappeared, the dose was increased. This cycle continued until, eventually, the child was referred for evaluation because the dose being given was so high. According to Segal's hypothesis (1978), these children were producing a compensatory response to counteract the drug effect and that may even account for the placebo findings, where there is deterioration of performance during the day. A compensatory response would impair performance after placebo, if that compensatory response is not counteracted with medication.

Dr. Bloomingdale: Did you give the matrix long-acting Ritalin?

Dr. Swanson: Yes, but we had real problems with the long-acting preparation in evaluating behavioral effect. We examined 15 or 20 children, and found no consistent response to the long-acting Ritalin. We have doubts about its effectiveness.

Dr. Hunt: As I understand your findings, those children who perform poorly on the paired associate learning (PAL) tasks may present two response patterns. Some may have improved behavior ratings in the classroom but perform poorly on the cognitive task, regardless of dose. A second group may demonstrate a dose-dependent effect. Their performance on the PAL improves on a low dose of stimulant but it deteriorates at a higher dose. As you observe these children in whom stimulants impair learning, are there any behavioral correlates of their cognitive deterioration?

Dr. Swanson: I think it is related to withdrawal, over-focusing, as described by Kinsbourne. Dr. Pelham used a code to evaluate these children and described their reactions, as they overdosed on pemoline, as: socially isolated in the playground at the same doses at which there are overdose effects. The over-focusing effect produces attention orientation to the task but not good performance.

Dr. Serfontein: We found a negative correlation between MPH and d-amphetamine in treating these children. Did you assess those children on high doses of MPH with d-amphetamine?

Dr. Swanson: We tried most of these children on pemoline and found good responses to low doses but thought we were also seeing tolerance because doses had to be increased to maintain effects. I think the tolerance may be learned, as Segal proposed. With pemoline once a day, a release from learned tolerance is observed, which then builds up again once a schedule is established. Switching to another drug may provide release from the tolerance.

Dr. Simeon: You mentioned that these children are started on an initial dose of 13 mg daily, which I think is very high. I never start children on more than 5 or 10 mg daily.

Dr. Swanson: I agree with you, but I was evaluating patients referred to me.

Dr. Simeon: I suspect that if they developed tolerance, they did so because they are on such high doses.

Dr. Hechtman: How do your findings relate to Dr. Gualtieri's in terms of serum levels?

Dr. Swanson: I used a task that shows a nonmonotonic effect. I think Gualtieri started to find that with the CPT but did not use a high enough dose. If he had looked at a task that required more effortful processing, he may have found a quadratic effect. There are no real discrepancies between our data; I used higher doses than they did. Some of the children were on a daily dose of 3-1/2 mg/kg.

Dr. Gualtieri: That's true; we found very strong dose relationships on virtually every aspect of performance, and they were generally monotonic. Whether another task would have revealed a different kind of response would require further experiments.

Dr. Swanson: But you had significant quadratic effects for the CPT, didn't you Dr. Hicks?

Dr. Hicks: Yes.

Dr. Quay: I don't believe you can say that you reach the ideal therapeutic dose with respect to teacher ratings because you are evaluating different effects, or factors.

Dr. Swanson: Sprague made the same point. The optimal, in terms of the lowest Conners rating, was at even higher doses. Sprague studied different ways of evaluating the optimal dose and maintained that emphasis on cognitive effect gives a better therapeutic response then emphasis on subjective ratings of parents or teachers. I concur completely.

Dr. Klorman: In some ways my findings overlap what you have been saying, while in other ways, they may not. There are two cautions I think should be maintained in discussing such data: (a) basically, it doesn't look like a quadratic trend when a slight quadratic effect is noted in a monotonic curve. Trend analysis is very sensitive to small departures from linearity, which may not have a great deal of significance, especially if they are carried by just a few subjects. (b) Your data include only three points, placebo, low dose and high dose. Expecially with a monotonic function, more points are needed to determine the best-fitting polynomial and the most reasonable order of that polynomial, taking standard deviation into account.

Dr. Swanson: We used five instead of three doses—placebo, 18, 37, 75 and 112 mg/kg of pemoline, in 28 subjects. The comments you made are correct. You have to worry about small groups and about two doses, but with five doses of medication and a problem as to what to evaluate, this is not a monotonic function.

Dr. Klorman: I observed a slight increment with one task and a slight decrement with the other, with individual patients, so the function was monotonic and not quadratic.

Dr. Swanson: My data are subject to the criticism that they are averages across subjects.

Dr. Pelham: We separated the children differently. We looked at the initial level of aggressive behavior observed in the playground and found very different patterns of response in social behavior for two subgroups. In observation of on-task behavior and a number of math problems the children did, we found linear trends for all measures in the same study with the same children.

REFERENCES

Barkley RA: Hyperactive Children: A Handbook for Diagnosis and Treatment. New York, Guilford Press 1981.

Bartlett RB, Egger E: Disposition and metabolism of methylphenidate in dog and man. Fed Proc Fed Am Soc Exp Biol 1972; 29:537.

Brown GL, Hunt RD, Ebert MH, Bunney WE, Kopin IJ: Plasma levels of d-amphetamine in hyperactive children. Psychopharmacology 1979; 52:133–140.

Brown GL, Ebert MH, Mikkelson MJ, Hunt RD: Behavior and motor activity in hyperactive children and plasma amphetamine levels following a sustained release preparation. J Am Acad Child Psychiat 1980; 19:225–239.

Burns JT, House RF, Fensch FC, Miller JG: Effects of magnesium pemoline and dextro-amphetamine on human learning. Science 1967; 152:849–851.

Chan YM, Soldin SJ, Swanson JM, Deber CM, Thiessen JJ, Macleod S: Gas chrome-tographic mass spectrometric analysis of methylphenidate (Ritalin) in serum. Clin Chem 1980; 13:266–272.

Chan YM, Swanson JM, Soldin SS, Theissen JJ, Maclead SM, Logan W: Methylphenidate hydrochloride given with or before breakfast: II. Effects on plasma concentrations of methylphenidate and ritalinic acid. Pediatrics 1983; 72:56–59.

Collier CP, Soldin SJ, Swanson JM, Weinberg F, Rochefort JE: The pharmacokinetics and efficacy of pemoline in children with attention deficit disorder and hyperactivity. Clin Pharmacokinet 1985; 10:269–278.

Conners CK, Eisenberg L, Sharpe L: Effects of methylphendiate (Ritalin) on paired-associate learning and Porteus maze performance in emotionally disturbed children. J Consult Psychol 1968; 28:14–22.

Dalby T, Kinsbourne M, Swanson JM, Sobol M: Hyperactive children's underuse of learning time: correction by stimulant treatment. Child Dev 1977; 48:1448–1453.

Faraj BA, Israili ZH, Perel JM, *et al.*: Metabolism and disposition of methylphenidate—14 C: studies in man and animals. J Pharmacol Exp Ther 1974; 191–535.

Gal J, Hodshon BJ, Pintauro C: Pharmacokinetics of methylphenidate in the rat using single-ion monitoring GLC mass spectrometry. J Pharm Sci 1977; 66:866.

Goodman L, Gilman A: The Pharmacological Basic of Therapeutics, 6th Ed. New York, MacMillan, 1980.

Gualtieri CT, Wargin W, Kanoy R, Kennerly P, Shin D, Youngblood W, Mueller R, Breese GR: Clinical Studies of methylphenidate serum levels in children. J Am Acad Child Psychiat 1982; 21:19–26.

Hasher L, Zacks RTR: Automatic and effortful processes in memory. J Exp Psychol Gen 1979; 108:81–89.

Hiscock M, Kinsbourne M, Chaplan B, Swanson JM: Auditory attention in hyperactive children: effects of stimulant medication on dichotic listening performance. J Abnorm Psychol 1979; 88:27–32.

Kausler DH: Psychology of Verbal Learning Memory. Academic Press, New York, 1974.

Kinsbourne M, Swanson JM: Evaluation of symptomatic treatment of hyperactive behavior by stimulant drugs. In Knights and Bakker (eds): Treatment of Hyperactive and Learning Disordered Children: Current Research. Baltimore, University Park Press, 1980, pp 207–217.

Kupietz SS, Weinsberg BG, Sverd J: Learning ability and methylphenidate (Ritalin) plasma concentration in hyperactive children: a preliminary investigation. J Am Acad Child Psychiat 1982; 21:29–30.

Laufer M, Denhoff E: Hyperactive behavior symptoms in children. J Pediatr 1957; 50:463.

Milberg RM, Rinehart KL, Sprague RL, Sleator EK: A reproducible gas chromatographic mass spectrometric assay for low levels of methylphenidate and ritalinic acid in blood and urine. Biened Mass Spectrom 1975; 2:2.

Pelham WE, Bender M, Wilson J, Swanson J: Paper presented at the American Psychological Association meeting, Montreal 1980.

Pelham WE, Schnedler RW, Bender ME, Nilsson DE, Miller J, Budrow MS, Ronnei M: The combination of behavior therapy and methylphenidate in the treatment of attention deficit disorders: a therapy outcome study. This volume.

Rapoport JL, Buchsbaum MS, Zahn P, Weingartner H, Ludlow C, Mikkelsen EJ: Dextroamphetamine: cognitive and behavioral effects on normal prepubertal boys. Science 1978; 199:560–563.

Schain RJ, Reynard CL: Observations and effects of a central stimulant drug (methylphenidate) on children with hyperactive behavior. Pediatrics 1975; 55:709.

Segal S: The role of Pavlovian conditioning in morphine tolerance. In Colpeart and Rosencrans (eds): Stimulus Properties of Drugs: 10 Years of Progress. Amsterdam, Elsevier-North Holland Med. Press. 1978, pp 325–350.

Sergeant J: Functional deficits in attentional deficit disorder? Chapter 1, this volume).

Shaywitz S, Hunt RD, Jatlow P, Cohen DJ, Young JG, Pierce RN, Anderson GM, Shaywitz BA: Psychopharmacology of attention deficit disorder: pharmacokinetics, neuroendocrine, and behavioral measurement following acute and chronic treatment with methylphenidate. Pediatrics 1982; 69:688–694.

Smith RG: Magnesium pemoline: lack of facilitation in human learning, memory and performance tests. Science 1967; 152:603–605.

Soldin SJ, Chan YM, Hill BM, Swanson JM: Liquid-chromatographic analysis for methylphenidate (Ritalin) in serum. Clin Chem 1979a; 25:401–404.

Soldin SJ, Hill BM, Chan YM, Swanson JM, Hill JE: A liquid chromatographic analysis for ritalinic acid [a-phenyl-a-(2-piperidyl) acetic acid] in serum. Clin Chem 1979b; 25:51–54.

Sprague RL, Sleator EK: Methylphenidate in hyperkinetic children: differences in dose effects on learning and social behavior. Science 1977; 198:1274–1276.

Swanson JM, Kinsbourne M: Stimulant-related state-dependent learning in hyperactive children. Science 1976; 192:1754.

Swanson JM, Kinsbourne M: Should you use stimulants to treat the hyperactive child? Mod Med 1978; 46:71–80.

Swanson JM, Kinsbourne M, Roberts W, Zucker K: A time response analysis of the effect of stimulant medication on the learning ability of children referred for hyperactivity. Pediatrics 1978; 61:21–29.

Swanson JM, Barlow A, Kinsbourne M: Task specificity of responses to stimulant drugs on laboratory tests. Int J Ment Health 1979; 8:67–82.

Swanson JM, Kinsbourne M: Food dyes and impairment of performance in hyperactive children: technical comments. Science 1981; 211:410–411.

Swanson JM, Kinsbourne M: The cognitive effects of stimulant drugs on hyperactive children. In Hale and Lewis (eds): Attention and Cognitive Development. New York, Plenum Press, 1979, pp 249–274.

Swanson JM, Sandman CA, Deutsch C, Baren M: Methylphenidate (Ritalin) given with or before breakfast: Part I. Behavioral, cognitive and electrophysiological effects. Pediatrics 1983; 72:49–55.

Swanson JM, Soldin SS: Serum levels and behavioral effects of methylphenidate. In preparation.

Taylor EA: Drug response and diagnostic validation. In Rutter (ed): Developmental Neuropsychiatry. New York, Guilford Press, 1983.

Thurston CM, Sobol MP, Swanson JM, Kinsbourne M: Effects of methylphenidate (Ritalin) on selective attention in hyperactive children. J Abnorm Child Psychol 1979; 7:471–481.

Tompkin CP, Soldin SJ, MacLeod SM, Rochefort JG, Swanson JM: Analysis of pemoline in serum by high performance liquid chromatography: clinical application to optimize treatment of hyperactive children. Ther Drug Monitor 1980; 2:255–260.

Varley CK, Turpin EW: Double-blind assessment of stimulant medication for attention deficit disorder: a model for clinical application. Am J Orthopsychiat 1982; 52:542–547.

Weiss B, Laties VG: Enhancement of human performance by caffeine and the amphetamines. Pharmacol Rev 1962;14:1–36.

9

New Generation Antidepressants and Attention Deficit Disorder

JOVAN G. SIMEON AND H. BRUCE FERGUSON

EDITOR'S SYNOPSIS

The authors started with the known therapeutic effect of antidepressants in the treatment of ADD and CD. They point out limitations, side effects and risks of both psychostimulants and tricyclic antidepressants. In the search for a safer and effective additional therapeutic agent, the authors present data from two studies: one on maprotiline (Ludiomil) and the other on bupropion (Wellbutrin).

The authors performed a 16-week clinical trial with maprotiline with 13 boys and 2 girls (ages 6–15) with enuresis and chronic behavior problems, including ADDH, CD, Overanxious Disorder and Depression. Enuresis improved in 14 patients (worsening in one), $p < 0.01$. Global severity of psychiatric illness improved markedly in 5 patients, moderately in 7, slight in 2 and none in the one borderline patient. Hyperactivity and sleep problems improved significantly but worsened at post-drug evaluation.

Fourteen ADD boys with hyperactivity and 3 with CD (ages 7–13) were evaluated in an open, single-blind clinical trial of bupropion. Clinical global improvement was marked in 5 patients, moderate in 7, mild in 2 and none in 3. T-test showed significant clinical improvement, as did the CPRS, PBRS-C, CTRS and Beitchman's patients' self-rating scale.

Adverse effects were infrequent, transient, mild and consisted of nausea or abdominal discomfort shown by eight boys. EEG showed significantly higher beta frequencies in the right hemisphere than the left at baseline. Peak beta frequencies converged between hemispheres with the drug. Greater clinical improvement with bupropion therapy was associated with: (1) lower peak delta frequency and lower percentages of delta amplitude at baseline and (2) higher percentages of alpha amplitude (especially in the left hemisphere) at baseline and during acute and chronic bupropion therapy.

The authors note that stimulants are generally more effective with classic symptoms of ADD, while antidepressants produce greater improvement in affectivity, sociability and self-esteem. These findings were consistent with their observations of the effect of maprotiline and bupropion.

This chapter regretfully was presented in summary form because of publishing requirements and the fact that bupropion has been withdrawn from the market. Copies of the original chapter may be obtained from Jovan Simeon, M.D., Royal Ottawa Hospital, 1145 Carling Avenue, Ont. J1Z 7K4.

10

Noradrenergic Mechanisms in ADDH

ROBERT D. HUNT, DONALD J. COHEN,
GEORGE ANDERSON AND
RUUD B. MINDERAA

THE DOPAMINE HYPOTHESIS OF ADDH

The dopamine (DA) hypothesis has been the dominant neurochemical mechanism proposed in Attention Deficit Disorder with Hyperactivity (ADDH) since Wender (1971) identified the role of DA in the control of movement and underscored the DA component of stimulant medications. Animal models of DA depletion following intracisternal administration of 6-OHDA to rat pups demonstrated increased levels of activity at 3–5 weeks of age and diminished performance on the shuttle-avoidance learning tasks; improvement followed administration of either amphetamine or methylphenidate (Shaywitz *et al.*, 1976a,b, 1978). However, CSF studies by Shetty and Chase (1976) showed normal levels of DA and its major metabolite, homovanillic acid (HVA). Shaywitz *et al.* (1977) using probenecid to block the egress of HVA from CSF, identified a modest decrease in HVA/probenecid ratio in ADDH children compared to children with other neuropsychiatric disorders. Pretreatment urinary excretion of HVA has been reported as normal (Wender, 1971). Furthermore, a therapeutic trial of the dopaminergic agonist, piribidil, did not appear beneficial (Brown *et al.*, 1979). In a recent trial, L-Dopa, in spite of being somewhat activating, did not significantly improve ADDH children's behavior (Langer *et al.*, 1981).

THE NORADRENERGIC SYSTEM

Several lines of evidence suggest a potential role for noradrenergic (NE) systems in the fundamental modulatory processes that include arousal, orientation, habituation, and vigilance. Furthermore, in recent studies, during the past 2 years at Yale, we have monitored the release of growth hormone in plasma following a single challenge dose of the noradrenergic agonist, clonidine. The pretreatment response of children with ADDH suggests the possibility of increased noradrenergic, alpha-1 postsynaptic receptor sensitivity in untreated subjects with ADDH (Hunt *et al.*, 1984). This increased noradrenergic sensitivity appears to diminish during chronic treatment with methylphenidate. Our recent double-blind placebo-crossover study of clonidine demonstrates a clear therapeutic benefit in the behavior of children with ADDH, both at home and at school (Hunt *et al.*, 1985).

Norepinephrine Anatomy and Physiology

The anatomy and physiology of norepinephrine (NE)—as illuminated by recent animal studies—suggest a central role of NE in the facilitation of arousal and attention and an enabling effect on the responsivity of other neurotransmitter systems. In contrast to the high degree of anatomic specificity in the organization of DA into well-localized tracts with more definable functions (Tassin *et al.*, 1982), NE cell bodies are located predominantly in the locus coeruleus (LC), from which they project extensively throughout the CNS (Amaral and Sinnamon, 1977; Aghajanian *et al.*, 1977). NE-LC axons extend to the spinal cord, affecting autonomic activity; they project throughout the cerebrum, modulating the activities of many types of cells, including the large pyramidal tract cells that centrally regulate volitional motor activity (Ungerstedt, 1971; Swanson and Hartman, 1975; Anden *et al.*, 1966). Indirect anatomic connections with the dopaminergic system occur via serotonergic interneurons (Bunney and DeRiemer, 1982; Anden *et al.*, 1976; Antelman and Caggiula, 1977). NE's physiologic effect on DA is evident from clonidine's reversal of the inhibition of dopamine firing in the nucleus accumbens of rats, which occurs during tail pinch or apomorphine administration.

The physiologic role of NE in modulating the sleep–wake cycle was identified by Jones *et al.* (1979), Foote *et al.* (1980), Ramm (1979). Recently Bloom and collaborators studied the spontaneous firing of the LC in unanesthetized, freely moving rats and monkeys (Segal *et al.*, 1976a,b; Aston-Jones and Bloom, 1981; Foote *et al.*, 1980; Foote and Bloom, 1979; Bloom, 1978). During the vegetative activities of grooming and sweet water feeding, the LC was quiescent. However, when a novel stimulus of light or sound was introduced, the LC abruptly fired. This LC activation preceeded and facilitated the action of other responding neurons to external stimuli. NE-LC activation produced a state of behavioral arousal and alertness characterized by increased vigilance and external focusing of attention. Increased NE-LC firing accompanied experiences of orienting, startle, awakening, and other sudden interruptions or changes in ongoing behavior; conversely, NE-LC activity diminished during the stable performance of repetitive activities. Thus, NE-LC firing facilitated a change in the level of arousal or in the response to environmental stimulation, which interrupts vegetative behaviors. Sensory-elicited discharge was accompanied synchronously by evoked field potentials from the LC, which may augment cortical or hippocampal resonse to the sensory stimulus (Segal and Bloom, 1976a,b; Gray *et al.*, 1975; Gray, 1982).

The NE-LC neurons are activated during transitions in behavioral states and participate in controlling generalized cortical and behavioral arousal. The NE system may not be involved in delivering specific messages as such, but rather may alter the state of neuronal circuitry so as to select between various synaptic inputs or between alternative behavioral responses. Activation of the NE-LC system facilitates the transitions between attentional foci or behavioral states; NE activation diminishes during states of sensory habituation or repetitive activity.

These two physiologic properties of the NE system may have important clinical relevance in ADDH. NE's diffuse anatomic distribution suggests broad physiologic modulation of the intensity and responsivity of many activities that may be transacted specifically through other neurotransmitters. Secondly, the activity of the noradrenergic system may be episodic, not tonic. Physiologically meaningful measures of NE must correlate neurotransmitter activity or release with specific behavioral or pharmacologic states. Single or baseline measures of NE activity may be misleading in a system that is episodically responsive and has a short chemical half-life.

Extrapolation of these noradrenergic mechanisms to man would suggest a central role of LC-NE in the modulation of processes of vigilance, arousal, and frustration tolerance. Inadequate NE activity may lead to impaired sedentary, contemplative, cognitive and emotional focus. It is precisely these behaviors that characterize the diverse symptoms of children with ADDH.

Animal Models of NE Depletion

Animal models of NE depletion have recently been produced through the administration of intraventricular, rather than intracisternal, 6-OHDA to rat pups. The relative depletion of NE compared with DA depends on the route and dose of 6-CHDA administered. These NE-deficient animals demonstrate a developmentally-transient hyperactive state (Pappas, 1980). Shaywitz *et al.* (1982) have induced NE depletion through intraperitoneal 6-CHDA in one-day-old rats. Although they became less hyperactive than DA-depleted rats, by day 19 both low and high doses of clonidine diminished their motoric activity; by one month, only high doses of clonidine retained this effect.

A cognitive alteration also follows disruption of the dorsal noradrenergic tract emanating from the locus coeruleus—called the dorsal bundle extinction effect (DBEE) (Mason, 1980; Mason and Iversen, 1978). Rats in which the LC is chemically or electrically ablated prior to learning under conditions of continuous reinforcement, demonstrate a delay in the extinction of learned behavior after the reward is discontinued. This phenomenon suggests that these rats are learning in a state analogous to intermittent reinforcement (which produces prolonged extinction). The noradrenergic deficit may produce a state of increased internal distractability during the learning phase.

Studies, at Yale, of externally-focused versus inwardly-directed attention in autistic and normal children have demonstrated a physiologic corollary to attentional direction that may reflect NE activity. During the execution of tasks requiring externally focused attention, such as marble sorting or visual scanning, peripheral vascular resistance increases and peripheral blood flow decreases (Kootz *et al.*, 1979). During internally directed tasks, such as mental calculations, the opposite physiologic status obtains. Individuals with type A personalities, who are prone to hypertension, also exhibit increased vigilance and noradrenergic tone. Thus, noradrenergic cardiovascular activity may parallel the degree of external monitoring.

Role of NE in Other Psychiatric Disorders

In addition to the long-standing interest in NE's role in affective disorders (Maas, 1974), at least two other clinical states may reflect increased NE activity. Gold has identified the noradrenergic component in opiate withdrawal—a state of heightened NE turnover and LC activation (Aghajanian, 1982; Gold *et al.*, 1980). Redmond (1979) has postulated that severe panic anxiety may reflect a hypernoradrenergic state physiologically identical to acute opiate withdrawal, which is transiently responsive to clonidine or to the beta-blocking effects of propranolol. Clonidine's therapeutic benefit in children with Tourette's Syndrome (TS) includes improved modulation of attention and impulsivity in those TS patients with attentional difficulties. In addition to reducing the tics, clonidine assists many TS patients to develop improved frustration tolerance and social adjustment (Cohen *et al.*, 1980; Leckman *et al.*, 1983).

NE Mechanisms in Children with ADDH

The NE metabolite, 3-hydroxyl-4-methoxyphenylethyline glycol (MHPG), is a useful index of NE metabolites in the brain, since 50%–80% of the urinary MHPG is of central origin (Kopin, 1978). Studies of urinary MHPG excretion in children with ADDH have produced contradictory findings. Shekim *et al.* (1979, 1983) have reported bimodal 24-hour urinary MHPG levels in untreated subjects with ADDH. Most ADDH children demonstrate diminished MHPG excretion compared to controls; a smaller percent excrete increased MHPG. Those ADDH children who had a favorable clinical response to d-amphetamine developed a further reduction in urinary MHPG excretion. Our studies in NIH also found decreased urinary MHPG excretion in amphetamine-responsive ADDH children (Brown *et al.*, 1981). In Chapter 11, Serfontein presents findings of decreased MHPG levels in ADDH. Kahn and Dekirmenjian (1981) reported increased urinary levels in dietarily unrestricted outpatients, compared to age-matched controls. Their data, however, suggest that the levels of urinary MHPG in children with ADDH were nearly identical to those reported by Shekim. However, their control group had unexplainably low urinary MHPG. CSF levels of MHPG have not been abnormal (Shaywitz *et al.*, 1977; Shetty *et al.*, 1976). Rogeness *et al.* (1982) reported diminished levels of dopamine-beta-hydroxylas (DBH)—the enzyme that stimulates the synthesis of NE from DA—in undersocialized children with conduct disorder.

Swanson (unpublished data) recently determined that a high percentage (about 45%) of children with ADDH do not normally suppress cortisol in response to a standard dexamethasone challenge. Since NE reciprocally inhibits corticotropin releasing factor (CRF), it is possible that ADDH children have either diminished NE inhibition, or that a tonically high NE state may reduce the response to dexamethasone challenge.

Interpretation of these varied individual measures of NE functioning is limited by the lack of concurrent measurement of receptor responsivity. In a chronic or steady state, low MHPG levels may reflect inhibition from hypersensitive, presynaptic alpha-2 receptors, or long-loop feedback inhibition from supersensitive postsynaptic alpha-1 receptors. Understanding of the neurophysiologic tone or responsivity of a neurochemical system, requires a research design that samples several sites along the neurophysiologic pathway (Hunt *et al.*, 1982). These measures might include metabolic and catabolic enzymes, levels of precursors, neurotransmitters, metabolite concentration reflective of turnover, and the activity of secondary messengers. A hypernoradrenergic state may be due to increased presynaptic production or release, or reflect heightened postsynpatic recetor response. An alteration in one component of a neurochemical system can be compensated for by changes in the sensitivity of another. Compensatory mechanisms may occur within and across neurotransmitter systems. Provocative tests utilizing agents with highly specific sites and mechanisms of action provide a controlled perturbation of targeted neurochemical systems. They enable monitoring of neurotransmitter systems in action and provide an index of neuronal responsivity and sensitivity (Hunt *et al.*, 1982).

Studies with the Noradrenergic Agent, Clonidine, in ADDH

Clonidine is an imidazole which, in low doses, is an alpha-2 presynaptic noradrenergic agonist. Iontophoretic and microelectrical studies demonstrate clonidine's inhibition of LC firing and its diminution of MHPG release (Cedarbaum and Aghajanian, 1976, 1977; Armal and Sinnamon, 1977). Given as a single acute dose in man, clonidine diminishes EPI and NE (Manheim *et al.*, 1982), decreases MHPG release (Starke and Montel, 1973), and reduces blood pressure, all suggesting a predominantly presynaptic effect.

Clonidine is a powerful releaser of human growth hormone (HGH), which is predominantly under noradrenergic control (Starke and Montel, 1973; Lal, 1975; Leckman *et al.*, 1983). Recent evidence suggests that the site of clonidine's release of growth hormone may be the alpha-2 presynaptic receptor (Cella *et al.*, 1983). Studies in unanesthetized dogs demonstrate that when the alpha-1 postsynaptic receptor is blocked by phenoxybenzamine or prazosine pretreatment, the growth hormone (GH) response to clonidine is unaltered (Anden *et al.*, 1976; Doxey *et al.*, 1977). However, pretreatment with the alpha-2 antagonist, yohimbine, which preferentially binds to the presynaptic receptor, blocks clonidine's release of GH, as does pretreatment with reserpine which depletes presynaptic NE stores (Cella *et al.*, 1983). This effect of reserpine-pretreatment in dogs is opposite to the earlier findings in rats. Species and dose differences in control mechanisms of GH release may account for this discrepancy.

THE CLONIDINE CHALLENGE TEST IN ADDH

We selected clonidine as a provocative agent in ADDH since it could provide a controlled perturbation of the noradrenergic system in children with ADDH. Our pilot study addressed three principal questions: (a) does the response to a single challenge dose of clonidine suggest an increase in noradrenergic receptor sensitivity in ADDH children compared to children with other psychiatric disorders?; (b) what effect does chronic treatment with methylphenidate (MPH) have on noradrenergic receptor response?; (c) is there evidence of chemical withdrawal one day after MPH is discontinued?

To enter the study, children had to score at least 2 SD above normal on either the parent or teacher rating of the Conners scales that was independently confirmed by two experienced child psychiatrists (RH and RM) using DSM-III criteria. The diagnosis of ADDH was established after standardized clinical interviews with parents and children, using their respective formats of the Diagnostic Interview for Children and Adolescents (DICA) by two experienced child psychiatrists. Behavior ratings were obtained from parents and teachers (Conners Behavior Rating Scales and the Achenbach Child Behavior Checklist). A brief neuromaturational assessment battery was performed with the child. Children were drug-naive and medication-free for 6 weeks prior to a baseline clonidine challenge test. Methylphenidate treatment was begun and continued for 3 months at a dose of 0.3–0.4 mg/kg/day. When titrated to optimal therapeutic response, 7 of 8 were rated as good responders.

The neurochemical response of 8 boys with ADDH (age 8–14 years, mean age 11 ± 2.2) was assessed following a single oral dose of clonidine administered before, during, and after the month-long treatment with MPD.

Procedure for Clonidine Provocative Tests

Diagnosed, consenting ADDH children were admitted to the Children's Clinical Research Center at Yale-New Haven Hospital. An 8-hour night-time urine specimen was collected prior to the provocative test and analyzed for catecholamines, MHPG and HVA. Following a regular breakfast, a 21-gauge gelco intravenous line was inserted into the non-dominant forearm and maintained patent with a slow, half-normal saline drip. Baseline measures of DBH, MAO, amines (NE, E, DA) and their metabolites (MHPG and HVA) and growth hormone (GH) were obtained after subjects were supine for at least 20 minutes. At 9.30 a.m., each child received an oral dose of clonidine (3–4 μg/kg). Sequential hourly blood samples for GH, amines, and metabolites MHPG and HVA were collected for 4 hours. Blood pressure, pulse and behavior were monitored. Not all subjects completed all phases of the study due to their reluctance to participate in more than two intravenous studies. Thus, these pilot data involve 4 to 5 children in each challenge test condition.

Response to Acute Clonidine Provocation

Before methylphenidate treatment, growth hormone levels rose from a baseline of 4.3 ± 1.4 ng/ml to a peak level of 31.3 ± 4.6 ng/ml at a mean time of 80 ± 8 minutes. This peak level was substantially greater than the peak GH response of children with Tourette's Syndrome (18 ng/ml), following similar clonidine provocation (Leckman *et al.*, 1984) or in children with short stature (peak level = 16 ng/ml). After 8 weeks of treatment with methylphenidate, a single morning dose of MPD (0.5 mg/kg) was administered at 8.30 a.m., 1 hour before repeating the clonidine challenge (Figure 10.1). Identical plasma samples were obtained for 4 hours after the 9.30 clonidine dose. In this during-MPH treatment condition, the GH response rose to only 14.8 ± 3.2 ng/ml, a peak level significantly (53%) less than that obtained before treatment ($p = 0.003$). During MPH treatment, the area under the curve (AUC) for GH released

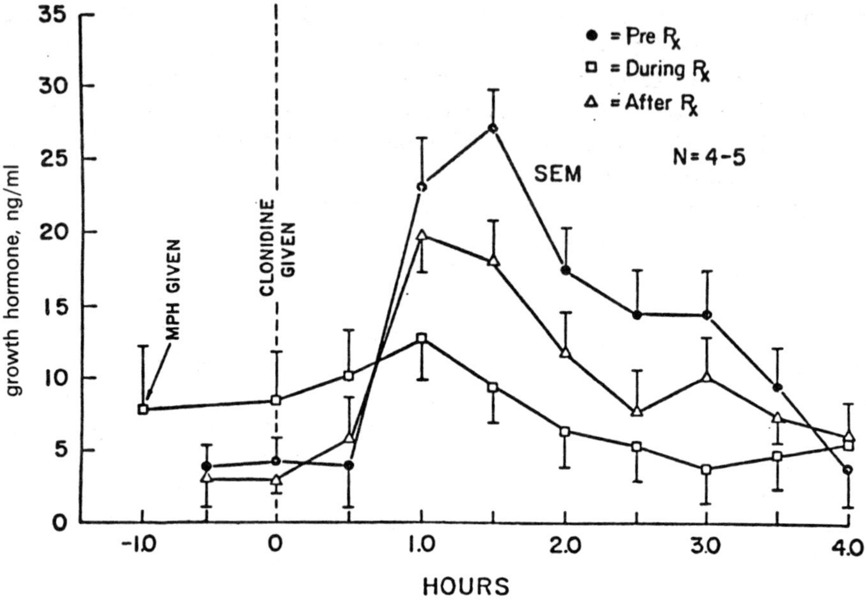

Methylphenidate (MPH) 0.5 mg/kg given orally at 8 a.m. to "During Treatment" Group.
Clonidine 3–4 ug/kg given orally at 9 a.m. to all children.

FIG. 10.1 Clonidine challenge before, during and after MPH treatment.

was only 1620 ± 353 mg/min compared to a pretreatment release of 3010 ± 823 mg/min. This was a significant decrease ($p = 0.027$). One day following the discontinuation of MPH treatment, the GH peak began to return to pretreatment levels, achieving a peak of 20.8 ± 3.9 ng/ml (66% of pretreatment peak) and an AUC of 2325 ± 623 mg/min (77% pretreatment levels): (difference in peak, $p = 0.04$; difference in AUC, $p = 0.08$). No withdrawal effect was noted, since the GH response 1 day after discontinuation was intermediate between the pretreatment and during treatment levels.

Concurrent measures of clonidine plasma levels demonstrated some decrease and delay in clonidine absorption during MPH treatment. Whereas before MPH treatment, peak clonidine levels rose to 0.98 ± 0.14 mg/ml at 80 ± 17 minutes, during MPH treatment the peak clonidine level was only 0.62 ± 0.01 mg/ml with a delay in peak time until 190 ± 29 minutes. Thus, following an acute dose of MPH, there was a decrease in the rate of clonidine absorption and lower 4-hour total AUC of clonidine in plasma. This suggests that MPH delays and diminishes clonidine absorption, however, this change in clonidine absorption does not fully account for the decrease in growth hormone response during MPH treatment. The correlation between peak clonidine and concurrent growth hormone levels varied significantly in each treatment condition. Before MPH treatment the correlation (peak clon: GH) was 0.81, while during MPH treatment the correlation between peak MPH and concurrent clonidine diminished to 0.32.

Further studies must clarify the extent to which the difference of growth hormone peak before and during MPH treatment reflects the combined pharmacologic effect of MPH and clonidine, or indicates a true, treatment-induced change in noradrenergic receptor sensitivity. Since both MPH and clonidine, when given separately, facilitate GH release, combined administration of those agents would be expected to diminish growth hormone release to less than their additive effect.

These results suggest an increased degree of noradrenergic receptor sensitivity in untreated ADDH children, which decreases during treatment with MPH. The exact site (pre- or postsynaptic) of this noradrenergic receptor sensitivity alteration in man requires further clarification.

MHPG Release Following Clonidine

A nonsignificant decrease in MHPG following acute administration of clonidine before, and 1 day after MPH treatment (12% and 19% respectively), occurring at 2.5 hours after clonidine (Table 10.1). During MPH treatment, the MHPG levels were suppressed further (baseline $= 4.53 \pm 0.23$ ng/mg, to trough $= 3.42 \pm 0.29$ ng/mg, a 24% decrease; $p = 0.01$), suggesting a greater inhibition of NE release during chronic MPH treatment. This reduction in MHPG may reflect diminished

TABLE 10.1

MPHG -- PLASMA LEVEL FOLLLOWING SINGLE DOSE OF CLONIDINE (3ug/ml)
Before, During, and After Methylphenidate Treatment

N = 4 - 5

	Baseline ng/ml	Trough Level ng/ml	% Change Base-Trough	Trough Time min
	Mean ± SE	Mean ± SE		Mean ± SE
Pre-Rx:	3.85 ± 0.36	3.38 ± 0.35	↓ 12 ± 2	150 ± 30
During Rx:	4.53 ± 0.23	3.42 ± 0.29	↓ 24 ± 14	132 ± 22
1 Day After Rx:	3.80 ± 0.65	3.43 ± 0.67	↓ 19 ± 12	135 ± 36
P-VALUES:	[DURING Rx:]	Baseline:Trough	p = 0.01	
	[% INHIBITION]	Pre-Rx:During Rx	p = 0.08	

presynaptic inhibition of NE during treatment or represent the combined pharmacologic effect of MPD plus clonidine.

Treatment Implications of Pilot Study

If a hypernoradrenergic state exists in children with ADDH, a functional noradrenergic antagonist such as clonidine might provide therapeutic benefit. Clonidine has been found useful in the treatment of Tourette's syndrome (TS), in which problems of attention and impulsivity coexist with motor tics (Cohen *et al.*, 1980; Leckman *et al.*, 1983). On clonidine, these children become calmer, less impulsive, and have fewer tics.

An alternative treatment is needed for ADDH, given the significant side effects and substantial incidence of nonresponse that occurs with stimulant medications. Anorexia, insomnia, growth retardation, induction of tics' sedation and personality changes—consisting of increased rigidity and diminished spontaneity with episodes of explosiveness—are important liabilities in MPH treatment (Greenhill *et al.*, 1980; Lowe *et al.*, 1982). Afternoon and evening withdrawal symptoms frequently disrupt families; the stimulant-treated child may be better controlled at school but behaves much worse at home. Recent studies by Swanson (personal communication) suggest that about 40% of ADDH children demonstrate impaired learning on a paired associate learning task following an acute dose of MPD or pemoline.

THE CLONIDINE THERAPEUTIC TRIAL IN ADDH

We performed both an open pilot study of clonidine in 7 children and a placebo controlled, double-blind crossover study of 10 children, ages 8–13, all of whom met DSM-III criteria for ADDH. Each child and his parents received a standard psychiatric diagnostic interview (DICA). Behavioral ratings by parents and teachers (using the Conners and Achenbach scales) and clinicians' ratings of DSM-III symptoms helped clarify the diagnosis and severity of the disorder. The final diagnosis was independently confirmed by two child psychiatrists (RH and RM). Baseline physical and neurologic exams and neuromaturational assessment were performed. Children were either drug-naive or drug-free for 1 month prior to participation in this study. The study design randomly varied the sequence of 4 weeks of placebo with 8 continuous weeks of active clonidine treatment. Biweekly behavior ratings were obtained from the teachers and parents using their respective Conners scales. Monthly assessment by clinicians included an interview, a repeated neuromaturational exam, and the clinician's rating of DSM-III symptoms. The neuromaturational exam included measures of fine motor coordination, attention span, visual scanning and impulsivity. Treatment with clonidine consisted of 4.5 ug/kg/day (usually 0.05 mg four times a day orally) for 8 weeks.

Results of Clonidine Treatment

Seven of the 10 ADDH children had a clearly favorable response to clonidine, as indicated by the teachers' and parents' behavioral ratings and the clinicians' overall assessment. Before treatment with clonidine, the teachers blind behavior rating (Conners 28-item questionnaire) was 49.0 ± 5.20 (mean, SE). During clonidine treatment, the biweekly teachers' behavior ratings demonstrated progressive improvement. By the end of treatment (8 weeks) the teachers' ratings had decreased to 25.79 ± 1.31 (Figure 10.2). This change was significant at the $p = 0.001$ level. Similarly, the teachers' hyperactivity index (Barkley, 1981) dropped from pretreatment levels of 1.99 ± 0.16 to 1.12 ± 0.06 at the end of active clonidine treatment ($p = 0.001$). When subjects subsequently returned to placebo, they deteriorated significantly.

Blind parental ratings documented a similar response to clonidine treatment (Figure 10.3). Parents' overall behavior ratings (Conners 48-item scale) declined from a pretreatment level of 66.85 ± 5.75 to 43.00 ± 6.29 after 8 weeks of clonidine ($p = 0.003$). Parents related significant improvement in the hyperactivity index (2.03 ± 0.16 to 1.34 ± 0.21; $p = 0.004$), in conduct problems (1.38 ± 0.16 to 0.99 ± 0.10; $p = 0.011$) and a trend of improvement in psychosomatic problems (0.26 ± 0.08 to 0.16 ± 0.7; $p = 0.025$). No significant improvement occurred in ratings of anxiety.

Clinicians' ratings also documented improvement in the clonidine-treatment children on their total score of cardinal DSM-III symptoms of ADDH. Assuming that a decrease in symptoms of 10%–25% is 'mild'; a decrease of 25%–50%, 'moderate'; and 51%–75% 'substantial', the children's ratings showed the following extent of improvement: inattention moderately improved in 4, mildly in another 3 subjects; and increased in one. Impulsivity improved moderately in 5, mildly in 3, and deteriorated in 2 subjects. Hyperactivity improved moderately in 6, mildly in 5, and one deteriorated. On overall clinician's ratings; 8 of the subjects improved, 3 substantially. Clinicians also reported that 7 of 10 subjects deteriorated in overall DSM-III symptoms of ADDH after switching from active clonidine to placebo (3 subjects could not tolerate the full 4 weeks of subsequent placebo). These ratings reflected an integration of clinical data which incorporated reports from parents and teachers with direct observations of the child.

While no significant changes were evident in the performance of neuromaturational tasks during clonidine treatment, the overall rate of performance tended to increase in tasks such as finger tap, coding, and

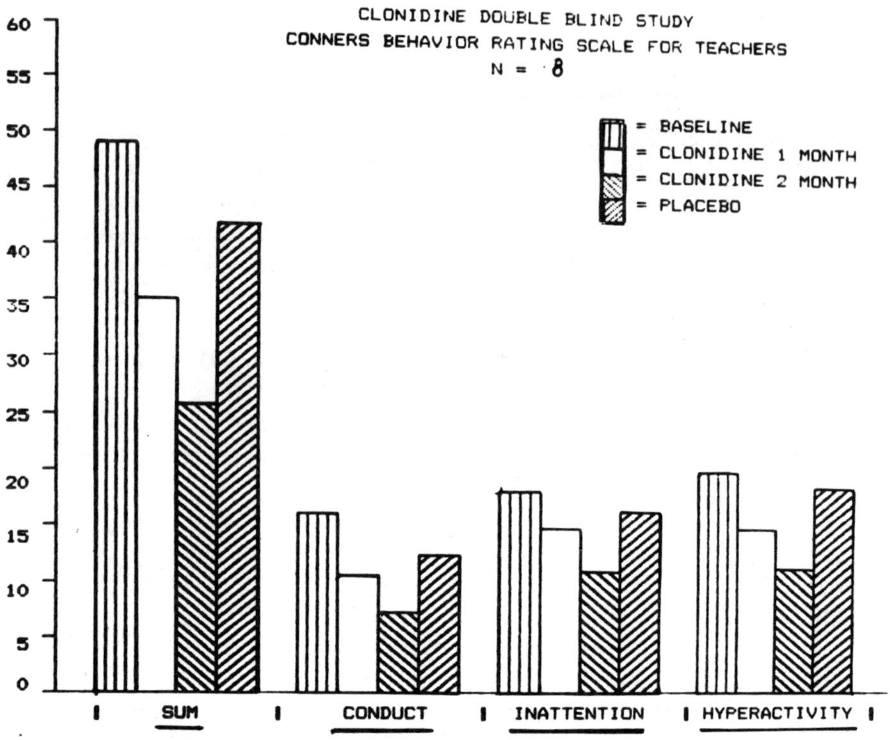

Factors for CONDUCT, INATTENTION, AND HYPERACTIVITY are multiplied by 10

p-values: line:	Baseline: Active (2 months)	Active (2 months): Placebo
SUM	0.001	0.05
CONDUCT	0.004	0.04
INATTENTION	0.09	0.05
HYPERACTIVITY	0.001	0.04

FIG. 10.2 Effect of clonidine on Conners Teachers Behavioral Rating Scale.

matching similar figures. Furthermore, there was a trend towards decreased variability in rate of performance. Collectively, these data suggest that clonidine is not improving children's behavior through nonspecific slowing or sedation. This reduced variability may suggest more consistent performance due to less distractibility and improved motivation.

Parents and teachers described these children as being "calmer, more compliant, listening better, and having increased frustration tolerance." Children were frequently considered to be "more mature," and "socially better accepted" during clonidine treatment.

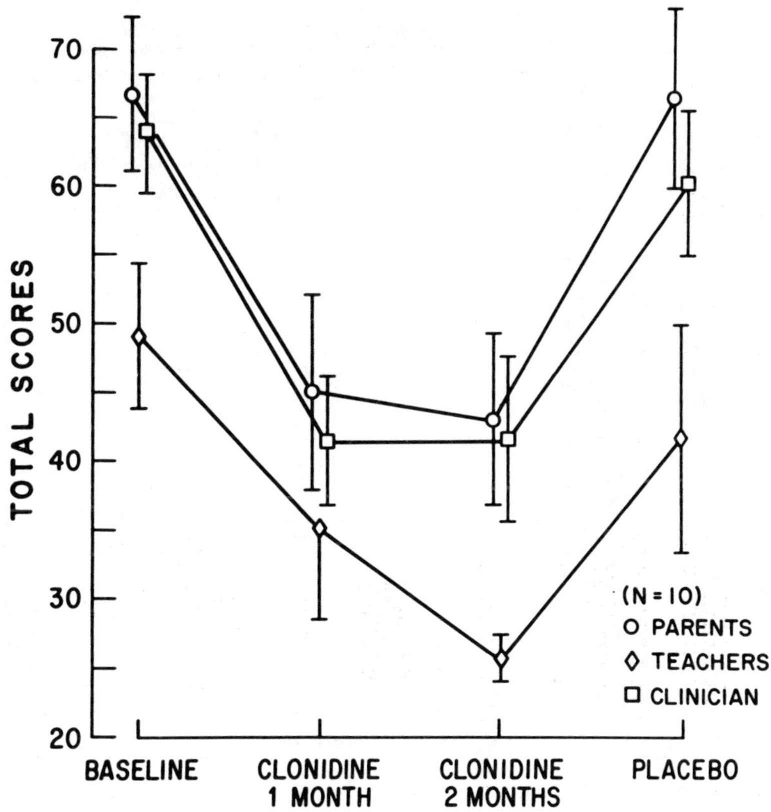

p-VALUES	PARENTS	TEACHERS	CLINICIAN
BASELINE : CLON 2 mo	0.003	0.001	0.01
CLON 2 mo : PLACEBO	0.02	0.05	0.04

FIG. 10.3 Clonidine effect on parents', teachers' and clinician's ratings.

The main side effect was sleepiness, which occurred for 30–60 minutes, beginning 1 hour after clonidine administration. In all but one child, this sleepiness subsided after 3 weeks. One child with a history of depression, again became depressed on clonidine. The two girls and one boy with schizoid personality disorder in the study were the poorest responders. In no child did overall behavior worsen. Most of these children continue on open treatment with clonidine; in some, a small amount of methylphenidate is now being given concurrently. This combination is well tolerated and may have additive benefit (Figures 10.4, 10.5).

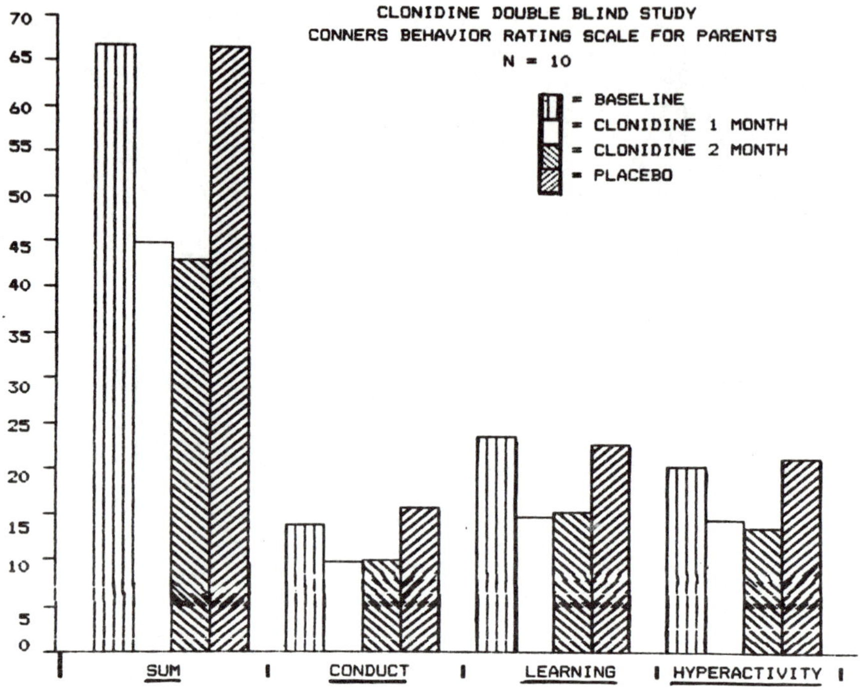

Factors for CONDUCT, LEARNING, AND HYPERACTIVITY are multiplied by 10

p = values:	Baseline: Active (2 months)	Active (2 months): Placebo
SUM	0.003	0.02
CONDUCT	0.011	0.01
LEARNING	0.007	0.03
HYPERACTIVITY	0.004	0.002

FIG. 10.4 Effect of clonidine on Conners Parents Behavior Rating Scale.

Clonidine appears therapeutically useful in a subgroup of children with ADDH. These children are being further characterized clinically and neurochemically. The relationship between GH response to clonidine provocation, pretreatment MHPG levels, and characterization of the differences in therapeutic response to clonidine or to MPH merits further investigation.

DISCUSSION

Homeostatic alterations in the noradrenergic system may mediate some symptoms of ADDH and coexist with shifts in equilibrium of NE and dopamine, serotonin, or other neurotransmitter systems.

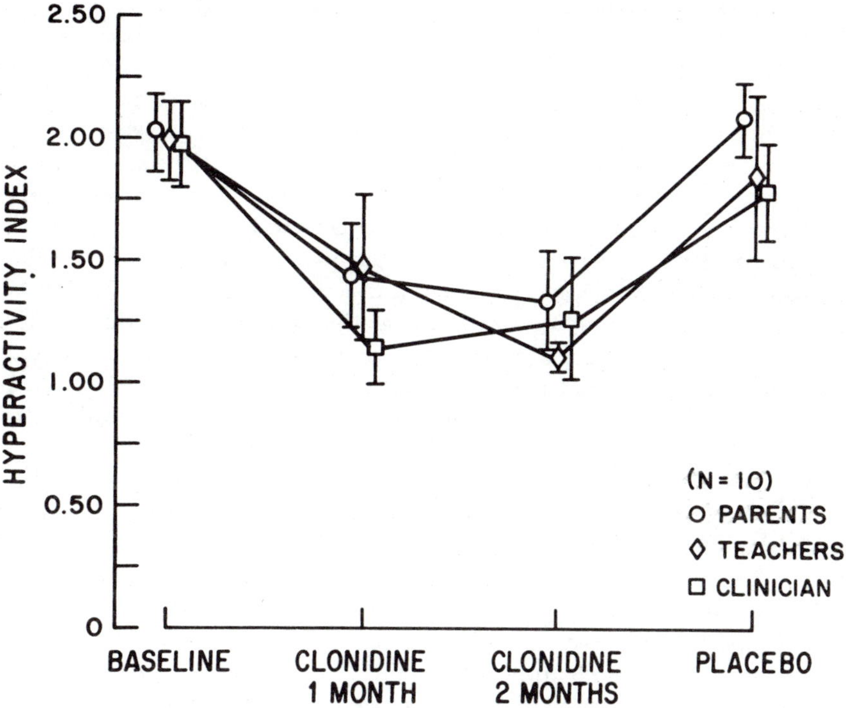

p-VALUES	PARENTS	TEACHERS	CLINICIAN
BASELINE : CLON 2 mo	0.004	0.001	0.03
CLON 2 mo : PLACEBO	0.002	0.04	0.12

FIG. 10.5 Clonidine effect on parents', teachers' and clinician's hyperactivity index.

The description of any clinical disorder as a hyper- or hypoaminergic state creates a semantic problem that implies a characterization of the overall status of the chemical system. The terms fail to differentiate conditions of increased neurotransmitter production from those of alterations in pre- and postsynaptic receptor sensitivity. These global characterizations obscure differences in initial receptor set-point, downstream or feedback effects, or in the homeostatic balance between various neuroactive agents (e.g., neurotransmitters, peptides, endorphins) that modulate the overall effect of the system. More specific terminology would discriminate a primary alteration in presynaptic processes of synthesis, storage or release (production) from a primary or compensatory shift in target receptor sensitivity or demand. Some symptoms may reflect a synthesis deficit, secondary to an inadequate supply of rate-limiting precursors or enzymes. In these conditions, neurotransmitter and metabolite levels may be diminished, while postsynaptic receptor sensitivity may become compensatorily increased. Alternatively, neural systems may demonstrate synthesis inhibition secondary to presynaptic (autoreceptor) hypersensitivity or to long-loop feedback inhibition from hypersensitive postsynaptic receptors; these may secondarily diminish the rate of neurotransmitter synthesis or release. A state of synthesis excess may derive from precursor overload or enzymatic overactivity. Synthesis acceleration may be driven by down-regulated auto- or postsynaptic receptors following receptor blockade or neurotransmitter deprivation. A functional imbalance or disturbance may occur at or near the synapse. Synaptic activation may reflect increased release (as with MPH), or decreased reuptake (e.g., tricyclics) or diminished neurotransmitter catabolism (e.g., MAOIs, decreased COMT). Synaptic reduction of neurotransmitter effect may reflect diminished release or decreased reuptake (e.g., lithium).

A neurotransmitter system that achieves homeostasis through a skewed balance between production and receptor sensitivity may be intrinsically less stable over a wide range of pharmacologic or environmental stressors. Such chemical instability may become physiologically evident as labile behaviors or symptoms during the extreme of activation. A state of diminished noradrenergic production and increased postsynaptic receptor sensitivity may become clinically manifest as a disruption in processes of habituation, focusing, vigilance, persistence, and inhibition. Such instability in the regulation of arousal and attention is the predominant characteristic of the behavior of children with ADDH.

Noradrenergic systems may be of particular importance as a final common pathway for many symptoms which beset hyperactive children. In children with ADDH, the principal site of disturbance may be in the rate of synthesis and release of NE or in altered synaptic receptor sensitivity. Our data suggest that the primary disturbances may occur in the alpha-adrenergic receptor. Whether the principal site of action is pre- or postsynaptic remains difficult to determine, since alpha-2 receptors are located at both sites and clonidine is active at both receptors in a dose-dependent fashion. Clonidine preferentially acts presynaptically but also stimulates postsynaptic receptors. If clonidine's stimulation of growth hormone release occurs primarily through the presynaptic alpha-2 receptor, as suggested by Cella (1983), this presynaptic receptor may be supersensitive in ADDH. Some children with ADDH have an increased GH response to clonidine, as noted in our pilot challenge study. This mechanism of primary pathology also would be compatible with Shekim's findings that a large subgroup of ADDH children have low levels of urinary MHPG excretion. Clonidine's therapeutic effect in those ADDH children who improve may consist principally of down-regulation of the sensitivity of the presynaptic noradrenergic receptor. Such a mechanism of action appears consistent with the slow onset and gradual escalation of improvement noted over several weeks of treatment. Clonidine's noradrenergic effect may also modulate the responsivity of DA systems. Studies of the effect of chronic clonidine treatment in a related diagnostic group, children with Tourettes's syndrome, demonstrated no effect on 24-hour urinary MHPG excretion but an increase in urinary HVA excretion (Leckman *et al.*, 1983). Clonidine's therapeutic effect may be mediated through changes in receptor sensitivity and/or compensatory alterations in affiliated neurotransmitters.

In a disorder as multivariant as ADDH, no unitary etiology is likely. In some cases a state of noradrenergic inhibition may exist which could predispose to episodes of excessive noradrenergic responses. Other ADDH children may have excessive NE production. Given the importance of noradrenergic homeostasis in the modulation of arousal and attention, a disturbance in either direction could impair attention. A flooding of stimuli may occur with insufficient adrenergic inhibition; an imperviousness to stimuli may be due to inadequate arousal. Both states could be behaviorally manifest by restlessness, inattention, and impulsivity in spite of their dichotomous levels on cortical arousal. The net behavioral effect of a pathologic or treatment-induced change in receptor sensitivity may also depend on the localization, or relative predominance of such a change in cortical versus subcortical brain areas. Hypothetically, other children with similar phenotypic symptoms may have a primary disturbance in DA systems, which effects activity; children with deficits in serotonergic modulation may have symptoms of attention disorder associated with aggression. Other unidentified neuromodulators or neurotransmitters may also be involved, either primarily or secondarily. Future studies may identify differences in specific aspects of cognitive functioning that reflect this variability in neurochemical pathology or treatment response.

The effects of clonidine and stimulants on behavior appear somewhat distinct. Clinically, clonidine appears to improve frustration tolerance, while methylphenidate principally reduces distractibility. These effects may be metaphorically considered to alter the signal-to-noise ratio of stimuli relative to intrinsic background disturbance (static) or to competing stimuli or distractions. Stimulant medications appear to enhance the strength of the signal, while clonidine may be diminishing internal background or noise. This metaphor, which is consistent with the clinical calming noted in clonidine-responsive ADDH patients, requires further testing using relevant cognitive paradigms.

No therapeutic agents, either stimulants or clonidine, are universally effective in ADDH—and no etiology may be universally pervasive. Our pilot data suggest that children with ADDH may have increased receptor sensitivity which diminishes with MPH treatment. They also appear to respond to the noradrenergic effects of chronic clonidine treatment, which may act principally through gradually reducing noradrenergic receptor sensitivity. Thus, the noradrenergic system may be a significant pathogenic site for the symptoms of many children with ADDH. Continuation of these studies will have heuristic and therapeutic value, especially as they are linked with further chemical, behavioral and cognitive characterization of subtypes of children with ADDH.

REFERENCES

Aghajanian GK, Bunney BS: Dopamine "autoreceptors": pharmacological characterization by microintophoretic single cell recording studies. Nauwyn-Schmmiedberg's Arch Pharmacol 1977; 297:1–7.

Aghajanian GK: Central noradrenergic neurons: a locus for the functional interplay between alpha-2 noradrenoreceptors and opiate receptors. J Clin Psychiat 1982; 43:20–24.

Amaral D, Sinnamon H: The locus coeruleus: Neurobiology of a central noradrenergic nucleus. Prog Neurobiol 1977; 9:147–196.

Anden NE, Dahlstrom A, Guxe K, Larsson K, Olson L, Ungerstedt U: Ascending monoamine neurons to the telencephalon and diencephalon. Acta Physiol Scand 1966; 67:313–326.

Anden NE, Grabowska M, Strombom U: Different alpha-adrenoreceptors in the central nervous system mediating biochemical and functional effects of clonidine and receptor blocking agents. Naunyl-Schmiedebergs Arch Pharmacol 1976; 292:43–52.

Antelmen SM, Caggiula AR: Norepinephrine-dopamine interactions and behavior. Science 1977; 194:646–653.

Aston-Jones G, Bloom FE: Norepinephrine-containing locus coeruleus neurons in behaving rats exhibit pronounced responses to nonnoxious environmental stimuli. J Neurosci 1981; 1:887–900.

Barkley RA: Hyperactive Children: A handbook for Diagnosis and Treatment. New York, Guilford Press, 1981.

Bloom FE: Central noradrenergic systems: Physiology and pharmacology. In Lipton ME, Killam KC, DiMascio A (eds): Psychopharmacology—A 20-Year Progress Report. Raven Press, New York, 1978, pp 131–142.

Brown GL, Ebert MH, Hunt RD, Rapoport JL: Urinary 3-methoxy-4-hydroxyphenylglycol and homovanillic acid response to d-amphetamine in hyperactive children. Biol Psychiat 1981; 16:779–787.

Brown GL, Ebert MH, Mikkelsen EJ: 1979; Dopamine agonist piribedil in hyperactive children. Presented at the 132nd annual meeting of the American Psychiatric Association, Chicago, Ill, May 12–18, 1979.

Bunney BS, DeRiemer S: Effect of clonidine on dopaminergic neuronactivity in the substantia nigra: possible indirect mediation by noradrenergic regulation of the serotonergic raphe system. In Chase and Friedhoff (eds): Tourette's Syndrome. New York, Raven Press, 1982, pp 99–104.

Cedarbaum JM, Aghajanian GK: Catecholamine receptors on locus coeruleus neurons: Pharmacological characterization. Eur J Pharmacol 1977; 44:357–385.

Cedarbaum JM, Aghajanian GK: Noradrenergic neurons of the locus coeruleus: inhibition by epinephrine and activation by the alpha-antagonist piperoxane. Brain Res 1976; 112:412–419.

Cella SG, Picotti GB, Muller EE: Alpha-2 adrenergic stimulation enhances growth hormone secretion in the dog: a presynaptic mechanism? Life Sci 1983; 32:2785–2792.

Cohen DJ, Detlor J, Young JG, Shaywitz BA: Clonidine ameliorates Gilles de la Tourette syndrome. Arch Gen Psychiat 1980; 34:1350–1357.

Doxey JC, Smith CF, Walker JM: Selectivity of blocking agents for pre- and postsynaptic alpha-adrenoceptors. Br J Pharmacol 1977; 60:91–96.

Foote S, Aston-Jones G, Bloom FE: Impulse activity of locus coeruleus neurons in awake rats and squirrel monkeys is a function of sensory stimulation and arousal. Proc Natl Acad Sci USA 1980; 77:3033–3037.

Foote S, Bloom FE: Activity of norepinephrine-containing locus coeruleus neurons in the unanesthetized squirrel monkey. In Usdin, Kopin and Barchas (eds), Catecholamines: Basic and clinical frontiers. New York, Pergamon Press 1979, pp 625–627.

Gold MS, Pottash AL, Sweeney DR, Davies RK, Kleber HD: Clonidine decreases opiate withdrawal-related anxiety: possible opiate noradrenergic interaction in anxiety and panic. Substance and Alcohol Actions/Misuse 1980; 1:239–246.

Gray J, McNaughton N, James D, Kelleyu P: Effect of minor tranquilizers on hippocampal theta rhythm mimicked by depletion of forebrain noradrenaline. Nature 1975; 258:424–425.

Gray JA: The Neuropsychology of Anxiety: An Enquiry into the Functions of the Septal-Hippocampal System. New York, Oxford Press, 1982.

Greenhill LL, Puig-Antich J, Halpern F, Sachar EJ, Rubeinstein B, Chambers W, Fiscina B, Florea J: Growth disturbances in hyperkinetic children (Letter). Pediatrics 1980; 66:152–154.

Hunt RD, Cohen DJ, Shaywitz SE, Shaywitz BA: Strategies for study of the neurochemistry of attention deficit disorder in children. Schizophrenia Bull 1982; 8:236–251.

Hunt RD, Cohen DJ, Anderson G, Clark L: Possible change in noradrenergic receptor sensitivity following methylphenidate treatment: growth hormone and MHPG response to clonidine challenge in children with attention deficit disorder and hyperactivity. Life Sci 1984; 35:885–897.

Hunt RD, Minderaa R, Cohen DJ: Clonidine benefits children with attention deficit disorder and hyperactivity: Report of a double-blind placebo-crossover therapeutic trial. J Am Acad Child Psychiat 1985; 24:611–629.

Jones G, Segal M, Foote S, Bloom FE: Locus coeruleus neurons in freely moving rats exhibit pronounced alterations of firing rate during sensory stimulation and stages of the sleep-wake cycle. In Usdin, Kopin and Barachas (eds): Catecholamines: Basic and Clinical Frontiers. Pergamon Press, New York, 1979, pp 643–645.

Khan AU, Dekirmenjian H: Urinary excretion of catecholamine metabolites in hyperkinetic child syndrome. Am J Psychiat 1981; 138:108–109.

Kootz JP, Gold JR, Cohen DJ: Social interaction and sensory intake rejection. Am Acad Child Psychol 1979; 18:462–479.

Kopin I: Measurement of neurotransmitter turnover. In Lipton, DiMasao and Killam (eds): Psychopharmacology: Generation of Progress. New York, Raven Press, 1978, pp 933–942.

Lal S, Tolis G, Marin JB, Brown GM, Guyda H: Effects of clonidine on growth hormone, prolactin, lutenizing hormone and thyroid-stimulating hormone levels in serum of normal men. J Clin Endocrinol Metab 1975; 41:703–708.

Langer DH, Rapoport JL, Brown GL, Ebert MH, Bunney WE: Questioning a dopaminergic hypothesis. Am J Psychiat 1981; 138:4,537.

Leckman JF, Detlor J, Harcherik DF, Young JG, Anderson GM, Shaywitz BA, Cohen DJ: Acute and chronic clonidine treatment in Tourette's Syndrome: a preliminary report on clinical response and effect on plasma and urinary catecholamine metabolites, growth hormone, and blood pressure. J Am Acad Child Psychiat 1983; 22:433–440.

Leckman JF, Cohen DJ, Gertner JM, Ort S, Harcherick DF: Growth hormone response to clonidine in children, ages 4–17: Tourette's Syndrome vs children with short stature. J Am Acad Child Psychiat 1984; 23:174–182.

Lowe TL, Cohen DJ, Detlor J, Kremenitzer MW, Shaywitz BA: Stimulant medications precipitate Tourette's syndrome. JAMA 1982; 247:1729–1731.

Maas JW, Dekirmenjian H, Fawcett J: MHPG excretion by patients with affective disorders. Int Pharmacopsychiat 1974; 9:14–26.

Manheim P, Paalzow L, Hokfelt B: Plasma clonidine in relation to blood pressure, catecholamines, and renin activity during long-term treatment of hypertension. Clin Pharmacol Ther 1982; 31:445–451.

Mason ST: Noradrenaline and selective attention: a review of the model and the evidence. Life Sci 1980; 27:617–631.

Mason ST, Iversen SD: Reward, attention and the dorsal noradrenergic bundle. Brain Res 1978; 150:135–148.

Millichap JG: Growth of hyperactive children treated with methylphenidate.J Leam Disabil 1978; 11:567–570.

Moore RY, Bloom FE: Central catecholamine neuron systems: anatomy and physiology of the norepinephrine and epinephrine systems. Ann Rev Neurosci 1979; 2:113–168.

Pappas B, Gallivan JV, Dugas T, Saari M, Ings R: Intraventricular 5-hydroxydopamine in the newborn rat and locomotor responses to drugs in infancy: no support for the dopamine depletion model of minimal brain dysfunction. Psychopharmacology 1980; 70:41–46.

Ramm P: The locus coeruleus, catecholamines, and REM sleep: a critical review. Behav Neurol Biol 1979; 25:436–448.

Redmond DE, Jr: In Fann *et al.* (ed): Phenomenology and Treatment of Anxiety. Spectrum, New York, 1979, pp 153–203.

Rogeness GA, Hernandez JM, Macedo CA, Mitchell EL: Biochemical differences in children with conduct disorder socialized and undersocialized. Am J Psychiat 1982; 139:307–311.

Seeman, P, Titeler M, List S: Dopamine receptors in brain and pituitary. In Collu *et al.*, Brain Peptides and Hormones. Raven Press, New York, 1982, pp 31–42.

Segal M, Bloom FE: The action of norepinephrine in the rat hippocampus: III. Hippocampal cellular responses to locus coeruleus stimulation in the awake rat. Brain Res 1976a; 107:499–511.

Segal M, Bloom FE: The action of norepinephrine in the rat hippocampus: IV. The effects of locus coeruleus stimulation on evoked hippocampal unit activity. Brain Res 1976b; 107:513–525.

Shaywitz BE, Klopper JH, Yager RD, Gordon JW: Paradoxical response to amphetamine in developing rats treated with 6-hydroxydopamine. Nature 1976a; 261:153–155.

Shaywitz BA, Yager RD, Klopper J: Selective brain dopamine depletion in developing rats: an experimental model of minimal brain dysfunction. Science 1976b; 191:305–308.

Shaywitz BA, Cohen DJ, Bowers HB, Jr: CSF monoamine metabolites in children with minimal brain dysfunction: evidence for alteration of brain dopamine. J Pediatr 1977; 90:67–71.

Shaywitz BA, Klopper JH, Gordon JW: Methylphenidate in 6-hydroxydopamine-treated dev. rat pups: effects on activity and maze performance. Arch Neurol 1978; 35:463–469.

Shaywitz SE, Hunt RD, Jatlow P, Cohen DJ, Young JG, Pierce RN, Anderson GM, Shaywitz BA: Psychopharmacology of attention deficit disorder: Pharmacokinetic, neuroendocrine and behavioral measures following acute and chronic treatment with methylphenidate. Pediatrics 1982; 69:688–694.

Shekim WO, Dekirmenjian H, Chapel JL: Urinary catecholamine metabolites in hyperactive children treated with d-amphetamine. Am J Psychiat 1979; 134:1276–1279.

Shekim WO, Javaid J, Davis JM, Bylund DB: Urinary MHPG and HVA excretion in boys with attention deficit disorder and hyperactivity treated with d-amphetamine. Biol Psychiat 1983; 18:707–714.

Shetty T, Chase TN: Central monamines and hyperkinesis of childhood. Neurology 1976; 26:1000–1006.

Starke K, Montel H: Sympathomimetic inhibition of noradrenaline release: mediated by prostaglandins? Arch Pharmacol 1973; 278:111–116.

Swanson LW, Hartman BK: The central adrenergic system. J Comp Neurol 1975; 163:467–506.

Tassin JP, Simon J, Glowinski, Bockaert J: Modulations of the sensitivity of dopaminergic receptors in the prefrontal cortex and the nucleus accumbens: relationship with locomotor activity. In Collu *et al.* Brain Peptides and Hormones. New York, Raven Press, 1982, pp 17–30.

Ungerstedt U: Stereotaxic mapping of the monoamine pathways in the rat brain. Acta Physiol Scand Suppl 1971; 1–48.

Wender PH, Epstein RS, Kopin IJ, Gordon EK: Urinary monoamine metabolites in children with minimal brain dysfunctions. Am J Psychiat 1971; 127:1411–1415.

11

Psychoeducational Correlates of Catecholamine Metabolites in Hyperactive Children

W. O. SHEKIM, R. GLASER,
E. HORWITZ, J. JAVAID AND D. B. BYLUND

EDITOR'S SYNOPSIS

Twenty-eight ADDH boys and 23 controls with WISC-R IQ of 80 or above had three 24-hour urine collections after two weeks off medication. HVA and MHPG were later assayed.

Each child received the following battery of psychoeducational tests: Wechsler Intelligence Scale for Children—Revised; Peabody Picture Vocabulary Test, Form B; Developmental Test of Visual-Motor Integration, and Wide-range Achievement Test. Several measures frequently used in the assessment of learning disabilities were also computed. Pearson Product Moment Correlation Coefficients were computed between each biochemical measure, each of the test variables, and chronological age. All of the data were analyzed with the Statistical Analysis System and a probability level of $p < 0.05$ was required for significance.

The authors listed the correlations of HVA levels with all the psychological variables. They concluded from the analysis of the differences between the mean that children with relatively low coding scores and relatively high vocabulary scores excrete high levels of HVA. It also held that the children with relatively high scores on the coding subtest and low scores on the vocabulary subtest excreted lower levels of HVA in the urine.

When HVA levels were compared with standard scores on the WRAT an analysis lead to the conclusion that children who excrete lower levels of HVA tend to be farther behind than children who excrete high HVA levels. The authors concluded:

> ... HVA-related findings (showed) that children who excrete low levels of HVA do not do well on the vocabulary, comprehension, digit span, and Verbal IQ on the WISC-R. They tend to do poorly on vocabulary and object assembly subtests relative to the means of the subtest. They also tend to do well on the coding subtest relative to the means of performance subtests. They

achieve poorly in reading, spelling, and arithmetic, they are behind in school, and their WRAT reading score is lower than their WISC-R FSIQ.

Correlations were also done between MHPG and the psychoeducational tests. The authors found that hyperactive children who excreted low levels of MHPG performed better on the block design and object subtests of the WISC-R and performed poorly on the comprehension subtest and Peabody IQ relative to WISC-R FSIQ. Children who excreted high levels of MHPG did better on the comprehension subtest of the WISC-R and the Peabody IQ but did poorly on block design and object assembly. Significant differences were found between highest and lowest biochemical quartiles within the hyperactive group of children in a variety of psychoeducational variables.

Regrettably Chapter 11 had to be replaced by this editor's synopsis due to publication demands and because a revision with reanalysis of the same data arriving at similar conclusions but in different terms has been published: Shekim WO, Sinclair E, Glaser R, Javaid J, Bylund DB: Norepinephrine and dopamine metabolites and educational variables in boys with attention deficit disorder and hyperactivity. *J. Child Neurolog.* 2:50–56, 1987. Copies of the chapter may be obtained from Walid O. Shekim, M.D., U.C.L.A., 760 Westwood Plaza, Los Angeles, CA 90024.

12

Neurotransmitter Metabolites in Children with Attention Deficit Disorder

G. L. SERFONTEIN, J. W. EARL AND L. J. JOHNSTON

Several studies have, in recent years, investigated previous assertions that attention deficit disorders (ADD) in children may have a neurochemical basis (Cantwell, 1975; Kornetsky, 1970; Wender, 1971). Most commonly implicated neurotransmitters are dopamine and nonepinephrine. Urinary methoxyhydroxyphenylglycol (MHPG) is a metabolite of norepinephrine reputed to contain a significant fraction of cerebral norepinephrine degradation. Maas *et al.* (1979) and Shaywitz *et al.* (1977) demonstrated that boys with ADD appeared to secrete significantly lower levels of MHPG than did their normal controls. Shekim *et al.* (1979) showed, in their study, that boys with ADD could be divided into two subgroups: (a) those who were clinical responders to d-amphetamine and also experienced additional diminution of their urinary MHPG with treatment and, (b) those who were clinical nonresponders and experienced no change in urinary MHPG values after treatment with d-amphetamine. Shekim and his co-workers (1982) confirmed their findings in a subsequent study and also pointed to the possible role of dopamine levels as measured by urinary homovanillic acid (HVA). However, Shekim's colleagues, in a separate study (Khan and Dekirmenjian, 1981), could find no difference between normal controls and boys with ADD in relation to urinary MHPG.

We were of the opinion that these conflicting reports needed to be clarified and the pattern of norepinephrine metabolism determined in normal boys and girls in an age-related study.

SUBJECTS

A local middle-class Catholic school was screened for all children between the ages of 5 and 14 years. Children in the top decile of their class academically, who scored five or less on the Conners Abbreviated Teacher's Questionnaire (CATQ) (Conners, 1969), were selected for the study as a normal control group. These children were further screened for no history of neurologic or psychiatric dysfunction. A total of 57 boys and 30 girls was selected.

A second group of boys only, of matching age range, was selected for having ADD. These children were chosen from schools with similar socioeconomic and academic structure and were in the same metropolitan region. Selection criteria included an attention deficit of 12 months duration or more, when tested on the Detroit Test of Learning Aptitude (Detroit Tests, 1967) discrepancy of more than 20 points between WISC-R (Wechsler, 1974) and WRAT (Jastak and Jastak, 1965) results; score of 15 or more on CATQ; and signs of soft neurologic dysfunction on physical examination.

METHOD

All children were subjected to a 48-hr diet free of biogenic amines, stimulants and preservatives. This was followed by a 24-hr urine collection, which was stored on ice using 0.5 g sodium metabisulfite as preservative. The ADD group was then given a 30 mg/24-hr dose of methylphenidate (MPD), and a further 24-hr urine was collected after a 24-hr interval. The ADD group was assessed for clinical response to treatment by a paired-associate learning task (Swanson and Kinsbourne, 1979).

Creatinine excretion was measured by the Jaffe reaction and total urinary MHPG (after hydrolysis of the sample to breakdown sulphate and glucoronide conjugates) was measured by capillary gas chromotography.

RESULTS

In the group of normal controls, urinary MHPG was found to increase with age according to the equation:

$$\text{MHPG} = 0.28\ (\text{age}) + 0.12$$

with MHPG in mmols/24 hr and age in years (Figure 12.1).

The increase in MHPG production with age was more pronounced in boys than in girls. In fact, younger girls (5–7 years) appeared to have much higher urinary MHPG excretion levels than did boys of a similar age. The level in boys increased more rapidly, catching up and surpassing the level in girls near puberty. When the MHPG value was divided by creatinine, there was no significant change in the MHPG/creatinine ratio with age within each sex group.

Comparison of the 52 boys with ADD and 57 age-matched controls revealed a lower mean urinary MHPG level in the ADD group than was present in the controls, viz., 0.31 ± 0.14 and 0.40 ± 0.27 μmol/mol creatinine, respectively (Table 12.1). A Wilcoxon test displayed a highly

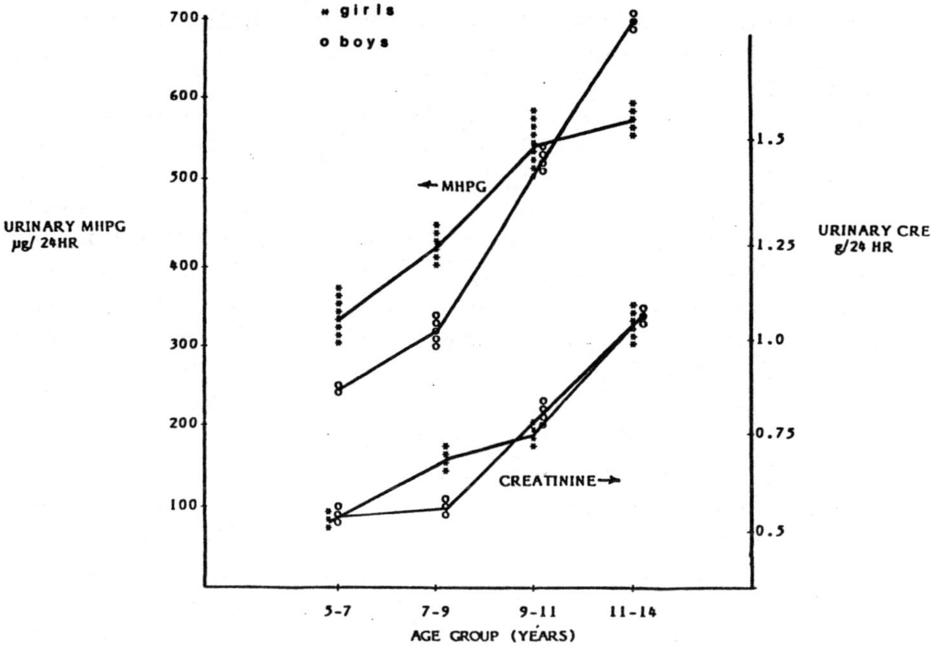

FIG. 12.1 Age Variation of MHPG and Creatinine.

significant difference between the two groups. When one viewed the number of subjects in both groups whose urinary MHPG was more than one standard deviation below the mean of the normal group, it was found that 16 in the ADD group and 2 in the normal group fell into this category. The ADD group was not normally distributed but skewed towards lower MHPG levels (Figure 12.2).

TABLE 12.1. *Comparison of MHPG in normal and MBD boys*

	NORMAL	MBD
Number	57	52
Mean MHPG (mmol/mol creatinine)	0.40	0.31
Range (mmol/mol creatinine)	0.13–0.61	0.01–0.68
Number with MHPG Less than 0.2	2	16

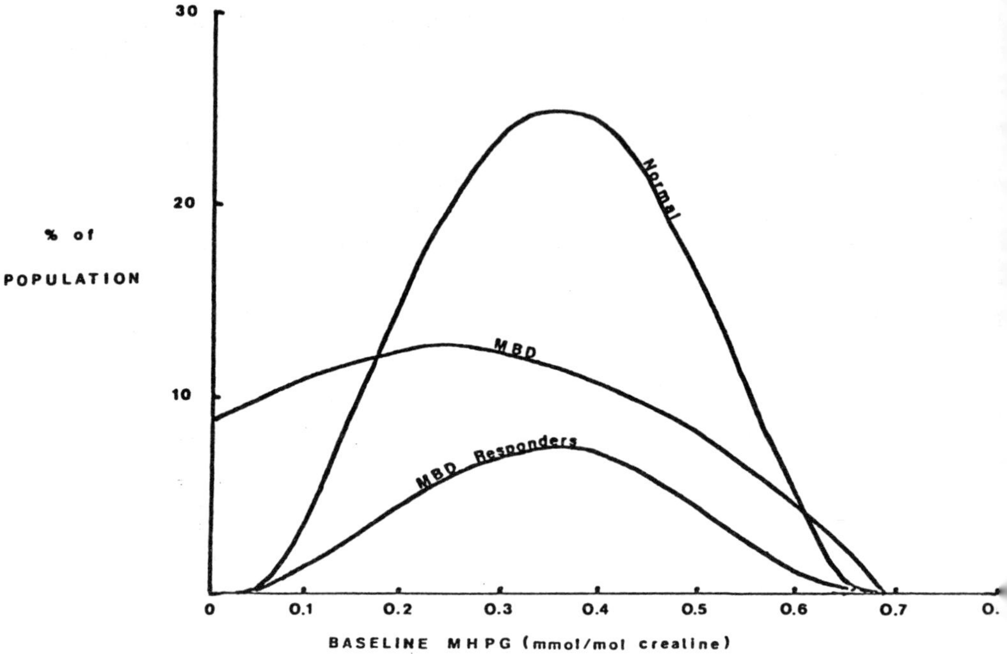

FIG. 12.2 ADD (MBD), ADD (MBD) Responders and Normals in per cent population vs. Baseline MHPG.

After the administration of methylphenidate to the ADD group, there was a significant decrease ($p < 0.05$) in MHPG levels in 31 subjects with a mean decrease of 0.17 ± 0.05. Using the criterion of 1 SD below the mean value of MHPG in the normal group again, we divided the entire group of 52 ADD boys into two subgroups:

1. The first subgroup had levels of MHPG above 0.2 μmol/mol creatinine, of which there were 36 with a mean value of 0.43 ± 0.19 μmol/mol creatinine. More than two-thirds were good clinical responders to methylphenidate and most of these experienced a significant decrease in MHPG values after treatment. The rest were marginally clinically improved, although half of these experienced a significant decrease in urinary MHPG after treatment.
2. The second subgroup had levels of MHPG below 0.2 μmol/mol creatinine. Of the 16 subjects in this subgroup, with a mean value 0.11 μmol/mol creatinine, half were good clinical responders to treatment but only a minority experienced diminished MHPG after treatment.

DISCUSSION

Our results tend to support the findings of Shaywitz *et al.* (1977) and Shekim *et al.* (1979, 1982) who demonstrated a significantly lower urinary

MHPG excretion in boys with ADD than in normal controls. Our data further support the work of Shekim *et al.* (1979, 1982) who showed that in boys with ADD responding clinically to methylphenidate. Methylphenidate urinary MHPG excreation was also reduced.

The ADD group could be further subdivided into two subgroups: the first group in which urinary MHPG excretion was within 1 SD of the normal controls; and a second group whose excretion was below this level. The first subgroup experienced a greater clinical response to methylphenidate (72%/50%) as well as a larger and more common decrease in urinary MHPG excretion after treatment (75%/25%) than did the second subgroup.

Psychostimulants such as methylphenidate and d-amphetamine are thought to potentiate the actions of the natural neurotransmitters, dopamine and norepinephrine, by increasing their secretion at the presynaptic cell and by inhibiting their reuptake into the postsynaptic cell. (There may be an effect of improving the affinity of the postsynaptic receptor site for binding with the neurotransmitter). The two groups of responders in our results lead to speculation as to whether there are not at least two types of ADD pathology: (a) a humoral and (b) a cellular. One could hypothesize that, in the humoral group, the psychostimulants may effectively depolarize the postsynaptic membrane but cause increased reuptake of the natural neurotransmitter in the presynpatic cell, acting almost like a false neurotransmitter which would lead to improved neutral transmission but with diminished metabolites for the true neurotransmitter. The cellular group with structural abnormality would have little capacity for this type of reaction.

This study contradicts the findings of Khan and Dekirmenjian (1981) in which they found no difference in urinary MHPG excretion between hyperactive subjects and controls. Our major criticism of that study was its methodology. Criteria for the selection of groups studied were "...boys known to one of us (AUK) and who were hyperactive." Similarly, the control group "...were selected from a middle-class neighborhood on the basis of their age and the willingness to participate in the study." All the results stand within the shadow of this selectional construct.

Interestingly, we could find no study that had included dietary control of biogenic amines during collection of urinary specimens, which is puzzling as the cerebral proportion of norepinephrine in urinary MHPG varies from 30% to 60%. The fact that we were measuring urinary MHPG as a metabolite of norepinephrine indicates that only one of the two known neurotransmitters involved in ADD was being investigated. Investigation of urinary homovanillic acid (HVA), which is the reputed metabolite of cerebral dopamine, may have added a further dimension to our study. Certainly, consideration should be accorded the fact that the clinical nonresponders to methylphenidate may have responded to d-amphetamine and possibly provided greater support to the humoral/cellular subgroup theories.

SUMMARY

Urinary MHPG excretion was measured in 57 normal boys and 30 normal girls. It was found that MHPG excretion was lower in boys until puberty, when it became higher than in girls. In 52 boys with Attention Deficit Disorder levels of MHPG, as a group, were lower than in the normal group, largely due to a subgroup with very low levels of MHPG excretion. ADD boys with more normal baseline MHPG responded better clinically to methylphenidate and also showed concomitant decreases in MHPG excretion after treatment.

GENERAL DISCUSSION

Dr. Pelham: What is the test-retest reliability for these metabolites? Is MHPG stable in a child a week later?

Dr. Serfontein: There isn't a great test reliability. However, in a pilot study of 10 children we found that the test-restest reliability was reasonable, although not highly consistent.

Dr. Swanson: Your data show that 34 of the children were good responders to the medication, and 18 were non or adverse responders. The percentage of children with decreased MHPG following MPD treatment was much higher in good responders than in adverse responders. These data suggest that changes in MHPG levels after treatment with stimulants may predict responses to medication.

Dr. Shekim: We found that responders had higher levels of MHPG than nonresponders and that changes in MHPG with d-amphetamine correlated somewhat with clinical response.

Dr. Serfontein: Although the precise data are not available as yet, it does appear that MHPG correlates with HVA, MHPG also increases in children who respond clinically.

Dr. Pelham: Why does the MHPG level become even more different from normal in children responding to MPH?

Dr. Serfontein: One can speculate on many bases that it stimulates dopamine release and also, perhaps, enhances receptors in the cell membrane, increasing reuptake. Therefore, metabolism in the synaptic cleft is slight. It may also act as a false neurotransmitter very successfully, which is another consideration.

Dr. Shekim: MHPG excretion is so variable that any difference observed by averaging three 24-hr samples will not be detected in a single sample.

In most studies reported in the literature one 24-hr sample was collected. At our center, we admit children for 7 days to a clinic research center with a very high ratio of nursing staff to subjects. The children are placed on a standardized diet and we make sure that they don't lose urine.

Dr. Hunt: Have either of you compared catecholamine levels in night time urinary collections to levels in 24-hr collections? I wonder if the night-time collection, which would control for level of motor activity, may be a more reliable and more replicable measure of MHPG?

Dr. Shekim: I wanted to compare 12-hr day samples with night samples, but Dr. Dekirmenjian, who was doing our MHPG assays said they had done this in adults and found no differences.

Dr. Serfontein: We made these assessments every few days and also after 3 weeks. As we could find no statistical difference between the two we opted for the more compact 4-day study.

Dr. Hunt: Effects of activity level on urinary MHPG excretion have been documented. Given the variation in the activity of the hyperactive child population, it may be important to compare day and night-time urinary catecholamine levels.

Dr. Simeon: What causes MHPG to increase with age?

Dr. Serfontein: The fact that it is pretty constant with creatinine would suggest that nervous and other body tissues grow at a constant rate as the child grows older.

Dr. Shekim: In normal children MHPG increases with age, creatinine and body surface. In our studies medication was discontinued for 2 weeks in children who were not medication naive.

Dr. Serfontein: Our children were all naive.

Dr. Simeon: After how many days on medication was MHPG determined and did you repeat the tests?

Dr. Serfontein: After 24 hr. In the pilot study, there was no difference between treatment for 3 weeks or for just one day.

Dr. Shekim: We found that body weight significantly affects metabolic studies. You did not report on body weight.

Dr. Serfontein: Like creatinine, MHPG is related to body weight and for this reason the MHPG-creatinine ratio is important.

REFERENCES

Cantwell DP: Hyperactive Child. New York, Spectrum Publications, 1975.

Conners CK: A teacher rating scale for use in drug studies with children. Am J Psychiat 1969; 126:884–888.

Detroit Tests of Learning Aptitude. Indianapolis, Bobbs-Merrill, Inc., 1967.

Jastak JF, Jastak SR: The Wide Range Achievement Test, Delaware, Guidance Associates, Inc, 1965.

Khan AU, Dekirmenjian H: Urinary excretion of catecholamine metabolites in hyperkinetic child syndrome. Am J Psychiat 1981; 138:108–110.

Kinsbourne M, Swanson JM, Herman D: Laboratory measurement of hyperactive children's response to stimulant medication. In Denhoff and Stern (eds): Minimal Brain Dysfunction: A Developmental Approach. New York, Masson, 1979, pp 81–106.

Kornetsky C: Psychoactive drugs in the immature organism. Psychopharmacologia (Berlin) 1970; 17:105–136.

Maas JW, Hattox SE, Greene NM: Neurotransmitter metabolite output by human brain (abstract). In Scientific Proceedings in Summary Form, 132nd Annual Meeting of the American Psychiatric Association, Washington, DC, 1979.

Shaywitz BA, Cohen DJ, Bowers MB: CSF Monoamine metabolites in children with minimal brain dysfunction: evidence for alteration of brain dopamine. J Pediatr 1977; 90:67–71.

Shekim WO, Dekirmenjian H, Chapel JL, Javaid J, Davis JM: Norepinephrine metabolism and clinical response to dextroamphetamine in hyperactive boys. J Pediatr 1979; 95:389–394.

Shekim WO, Javaid J, Dekirmenjian H, Chapel JL, Davis JM: Effects of d-amphetamine on urinary metabolites of dopamine and norepinephrine in hyperactive boys. Am J Psychiat 1982; 139:485–488.

Swanson JM, Kinsbourne M: Laboratory measurement of attention. In Denhoff and Stern (eds): Minimal Brain Dysfunction: A Developmental Approach. New York, Masson, 1979

Wechsler D: Manual for the Wechsler Intelligence Scale for Children—Revised. New York, The Psychological Corporation, 1974.

Wender PH: Minimal Brain Dysfunction in Children. New York, John Wiley and Sons, 1971.

13

Conners' Teacher Rating Scale: Reliability, Validity and Normative Data

RONALD L. TRITES

EDITOR'S SYNOPSIS

The author summarized in this chapter the result of a series of analyses of the reliability, validity, profile interpretation and normative investigation of the Conners Teacher Rating Scale (CTRS). Much of the data used for these analyses came from a prevalence study conducted with a randomly selected sample of 14,083 school children in Ottawa, Canada from 1970 to 1978 (Trites, 1979).

1,154 children were taught daily by an English language teacher in the morning and a French language teacher in the afternoon. Both teachers rated the children on the CTRS independently and the inter-rater agreement was found to be highly significant (p 0.001) for all factors (Trites *et al.*, 1981). 1,107 children were assessed one year later by a different teacher on the CTRS and again correlation of Conners original four factors were highly significant (p 0.0001). However, it was noted that only half of the children obtained scores above the cut-off (1.5) on the first testing retained it on the second rating. The author found there was a much higher referral rate to school psychologists of children who exceeded the cut-off on one or more of the factor scores than matched controls, especially among boys.

Dr. Trites performed a factor analysis of his large series (Trites *et al.*, 1982) and established a new factor structure found to be congruent between random half samples. Norms for a six-factor scoring system were established for ages 4–12 (Trites *et al.*, 1982). The author concludes that there is an independent syndrome of hyperactivity. 1.6 percent of the children obtained a score above the cut-off on the hyperactivity factor but were below cut-off on the remaining five factors (agreeing with Rutter's Isle of Wight figure). All children above cut-off on the hyperactivity factor led to a prevalence rate of 5.7% agreeing with other estimates in the literature.

We regret that Dr. Trites' chapter had to be summarized for reasons of publication and because the findings in his Chapter are available in the list of references. A copy of his Chapter may be obtained from Ronald L. Trites, Ph.D., Neuropsychology Laboratory, Royal Ottawa Hospital, 1145 Carling, Ottawa, Ontario K1Z 7K4, Canada.

REFERENCES

Trites RL: Prevalence of hyperactivity in the Ottawa-Carleton region. In Trites (Ed.): Hyperactivity in Children: Etiology, Measurement and Treatment Implication. Baltimore: University Park Press, 1979.

Trites RL, Blouin AGA, Ferguson HB, Lynch GW: The Conners Teacher Rating Scale: an epidemiologic inter-rater reliability and follow-up investigation. In K. Gadow and J. Loney (eds): Psychosocial Aspects of Drug Treatment for Hyperactivity. Chapt. 4, AAAS, Westview Press, 1981, pp 151–175.

Trites RL, Laprade K, Blouin AGA: Factor analysis of the Conners Teacher Rating Scale based on a large normative sample. J Consult Clin Psychol 1982; 50:615–623.

14

Reliability and Principal Component Analysis (PCA) of the Conners Teacher Questionnaire (CTQ)

JACQUES THIVIERGE,
MAURICE BOUDREAULT AND MICHEL MAZIADE

This paper focuses on some reliability and Principal Component Analysis (PCA) aspects of the Conners Teacher Questionnnaire (CTQ). Discussed are primarily: (a) the test–retest (T–R) reliability of the factors obtained through PCA, with and without rotation, and (b) the consequences of the reliability aspects in the interpretation of the factors.

METHODOLOGY

The Early Clinical Drug Evaluation Unit (ECDEU, 1976) version of the CTQ, translated by us into French, was administered twice to a non-clinical, random sample of 859 of the 6250 second-grade child population of the metropolitan Quebec City area, a French-speaking community.

Table 14.1 shows the elementary statistical description of the sample. Each teacher evaluated pupils on the CTQ originally and after a 3-week interval.

RESULTS

T–R Reliability of the Questions

"A question is said to be reliable if it reproduces within a relatively short interval of time the same results when applied to the same subject" (Magnusson, 1967). So defined, the reliability of the question cannot be appropriately assessed by a Pearson Correlation Coefficient. Therefore, we used a more straightforward approach: For each sample individual and for every question we computed the difference in absolute value of the

TABLE 14.1

Statistical Description of the Sample (N = 859)

Age:	Mean	7.8 years old
	Median	7.5 years old
Sex:	Girls	421 (49%)
	Boys	438 (51%)

Socio-Economic Classes (Hollingshead Two-Factor)

Class I	8.3%
Class II	9.1%
Class III	24.4%
Class IV	34.7%
Class V	23.5%

response to the test and to the retest. The difference noted, Δ_{ij}, is the numerical difference between the two ratings for the individual i, to the question j. Since we cannot, realistically, expect exact replication of the score from one rating to the other, we chose an arbitrary proportion of each possible value of Δ_{ij}, beyond which a question was considered reliable and unreliable.

A statistical test (Klotz, 1978) was performed to verify the reliability of every question according to this criterion. Two questions were found unreliable: 9 and 37.

T–R Reliability of the Factors

Four PCA were run, with and witout rotation, on both test and retest. In these four analyses, seven factors showed up with a variance >1. Table 14.2 shows the results of PCA on one of these four analyses.

(a) First, what might be termed a pure mathematical approach: We considered the 39 items of a factor; the factor will be said to be reliable if the T–R difference between "the square root of the relative contribution of the items to the factors" is <0.03 for all, or almost all, of its items. The relative contribution (RC) is the loading (1) of item i on the factor j (1_{ij}) divided by the contribution of the factor. Practically speaking, this means

TABLE 14.2

Reliability Criterion on Items

Possible Score Differences Between Test (January) and Retest (February)	Chosen Level of Reliability for Each Question

TABLE 14.3

UNROTATED FACTOR MATRIX, EIGENVALUES AND PERCENTAGE OF VARIANCE (JANUARY)

ITEMS	F-1	F-2	F-3	F-4	F-5	F-6	F-7	COMMUNALITY
1. Fidgeting	.73	-.25	-.27	.28	-.06	.19	-.04	.79
2. Hums	.67	-.16	-.09	.23	-.08	.18	-.20	.62
3. Demands	.64	- 0	.28	.28	-.07	-.08	.19	.62
4. Coordination	.34	.55	-.17	.05	.06	-.05	.08	.46
5. Restless	.69	-.29	-.18	.28	.01	.26	-.10	.75
6. Excitable	.75	-.17	-.09	.32	-.08	.14	-.08	.74
7. Inattentive	.65	.23	-.43	.19	-.07	-.13	.20	.75
8. Short span	.57	.29	-.36	.09	-.01	-.20	.31	.68
9. Sensitive	.18	.24	.53	.35	.15	.11	.06	.54
10. Serious	.14	.50	.26	-.06	-.08	.01	-.36	.48
11. Daydreams	.39	.52	-.18	.17	-.06	-.33	-.06	.60
12. Sullen	.67	.14	.32	-.06	-.27	-.12	-.15	.69
13. Cries	.30	.33	.32	.15	-.47	.10	.19	.59
14. Disturbs	.77	-.25	-.29	.14	-.03	.15	-.04	.78
15. Quarrelsome	.81	-.12	-.01	-.12	-.10	.07	-.03	.70
16. Moods	.70	.08	.33	.08	-.33	-.09	-.06	.74
17. Acts smart	.51	-.08	.24	.26	.32	-.01	-.08	.50
18. Destructive	.65	-.06	.07	-.34	-.02	.26	.08	.63
19. Steals	.45	.04	.09	-.48	-.08	.26	.29	.60
20. Lies	.61	.03	.06	-.38	-.04	.12	.30	.63
21. Temper	.64	.04	.31	-.11	-.36	-.01	.15	.68
22. Isolates	.11	.60	.03	-.02	-.08	-.22	-.27	.50
23. Unaccepted	.49	.34	.03	-.33	.19	-.11	-.11	.53
24. Easily led	-.01	.71	-.33	.06	.01	.19	.10	.66
25. No fair play	.69	.03	.01	-.25	.25	.03	.08	.62
26. Leadership	.14	.73	-.27	-.06	.03	.11	.02	.65
27. Opposite sex	.65	.10	.11	-.23	.35	-.02	-.17	.64
28. Same sex	.71	.05	.03	-.25	.26	.01	-.11	.65
29. Teases	.77	-.17	-.24	.04	.03	.16	-.06	.71
30. Submissive	-.49	.21	.15	.09	.25	.34	.09	.50
31. Defiant	.73	-.17	.05	-.07	.19	-.02	-.15	.63
32. Impudent	.66	-.14	.07	-.07	.12	0	-.18	.51
33. Shy	-.22	.74	.01	.03	.01	.26	-.08	.68
34. Fearful	-.18	.73	.06	.09	- 0	.37	-.13	.74
35. Excessive	.67	.14	0	.21	.24	-.17	.16	.63
36. Stubborn	.72	-.05	.19	-.05	-.08	-.14	-.03	.58
37. Anxious	-.06	.06	.49	.35	.44	.04	.31	.66
38. Uncooperative	.52	.12	-.01	-.07	.23	-.16	.04	.37
39. Attendance	.22	.19	-.02	.03	.10	-.28	.13	.19
Eigenvalue:	12.30	4.28	2.06	1.73	1.43	1.17	1.03	
% of variance:	.32	.11	.06	.04	.04	.03	.03	
$l_o = \sqrt{\frac{\lambda}{39}}$	.56	.33	.23	.21	.19	.17	.16	

TABLE 14.4

TEST-RETEST RELIABILITY OF UNROTATED FACTORS BASED ON THE DIFFERENCE

BETWEEN RELATIVE CONTRIBUTIONS (R.C.) OF ITEMS

ITEMS	F-1	F-2	F-3	F-4	F-5	F-6	F-7
1. Fidgeting	0	0	.08*	.09	.03	.19	.19
2. Hums	0	.03	.05	.11	.16	.35	.19
3. Demands	.01	.01	.10	.10	.09	.04	.15
4. Coordination	.01	0	0	.01	.07	.08	.26
5. Restless	.01	.01	.07	.10	.03	.25	.30
6. Excitable	0	.01	.11	.15	.03	.20	.26
7. Inattentive	0	.02	.03	.20	.18	.17	.23
8. Short span	0	.01	.04	.13	.33	.32	.42
9. Sensitive	.01	.03	.22	.13	.14	.15	.13
10. Serious	.01	.01	.02	.03	.13	.27	.31
11. Daydreams	.01	0	.05	.08	.10	.17	.15
12. Sullen	.01	.01	.02	.06	.17	.18	.13
13. Cries	.01	.01	.09	.08	.08	.35	.04
14. Disturbs	0	.01	.03	.12	.02	.13	.18
15. Quarrelsome	0	.03	.01	.03	.24	.08	.09
16. Moods	.01	.01	0	.05	.13	.13	.14
17. Acts smart	.02	.02	.08	.02	.16	.05	.03
18. Destructive	.01	.02	.12	.11	.07	.15	.01
19. Steals	.02	0	.18	.12	.11	.05	.14
20. Lies	.01	.02	.18	.09	.10	.26	.21
21. Temper	.01	.04	.05	.03	.19	0	.03
22. Isolates	.01	.01	0	.13	.01	.06	.10
23. Unaccepted	.02	.03	.05	.14	.01	.02	.20
24. Easily led	.02	.01	.04	.07	.10	.04	.09
25. No fair play	.01	.02	.13	.03	.17	.23	.12
26. Leadership	0	.01	.03	.02	.07	.06	.05
27. Opposite sex	0	.01	.02	.16	.11	.07	.06
28. Same sex	.01	.01	0	.09	.20	.08	.02
29. Teases	0	.01	.03	.11	.17	.10	.16
30. Submissive	.01	.02	.01	.16	.07	.09	.09
31. Defiant	0	.03	.05	.07	0	.05	.15
32. Impudent	.02	0	.10	.07	.13	.02	.19
33. Shy	.02	.01	0	.07	.13	.22	.35
34. Fearful	.04	.01	.01	.06	.16	.32	.47
35. Excessive	.01	.02	.07	.15	.28	.35	.22
36. Stubborn	.01	.01	.03	.01	.01	.14	.03
37. Anxious	0	.01	.13	.23	.28	.18	.49
38. Uncooperative	.01	.01	.01	.19	.23	.49	.33
39. Attendance	.02	.04	.09	.10	.16	.24	.38
Number of unstable items	1	2	22	31	31	36	34

* Measure of the difference between test-retest $\sqrt{R.C.}$ is greater than .03

that we standardized every factor and specified that the T–R difference on the questions be no more than 0.03. Using this criterion, as shown in Table 14.3, with the unrotated method only the first two factors are reliable. Applying the same criteria to the rotated data with seven factors, only the first one is reliable from test to retest.

(b) Our second method of examining the test–retest reliability of the factors utilized a more usual procedure (Table 14.4). We considered only the questions having high loading on the factors; in this approach, a factor will be said to be reliable if the questions contributing the most variance to the test are also those on the retest. If we look at the unrotated data

(Table 14.5), only the first two factors are reliable also; additionally, one can observe on this table that the greater the variance on a factor, the greater its reliability and the less its variance, the less its reliability. Examining the rotated data (Table 14.6) one can observe that the most reliable factor is the fourth, i.e., fourth in importance in terms of the explained variance. This mathematical procedure created an instability in the most important factor determined by the PCA method. As rotation can be performed on various factors, we asked ourselves what would happen to the test–retest reliability of a factor if we executed the rotation with a different number of factors. Table 14.7 shows the effect on the test–retest reliability of Factor I when we successively rotated 4, 5, 6 and 7 factors;

TABLE 14.5

TEST-RETEST RELIABILITY OF ROTATED FACTORS BASED ON THE DIFFERENCE BETWEEN RELATIVE CONTRIBUTIONS (R.C.) OF ITEMS

ITEMS	F-1	F-2	F-3	F-4	F-5	F-6	F-7
1. Fidgeting	.01	.03	0	.02	.05	.07	.11
2. Hums	.06*	.05	.03	.06	.09	.12	.06
3. Demands	.01	.02	0	.09	.23	.03	.26
4. Coordination	0	.06	.04	.06	.05	.03	.04
5. Restless	.02	0	.01	.02	.01	.02	.09
6. Excitable	.01	.01	0	.04	.09	.06	0
7. Inattentive	.03	.01	.03	.03	.13	.12	.04
8. Short span	.02	.05	.04	.02	.17	.12	.12
9. Sensitive	.01	.02	.07	.02	.17	.23	.25
10. Serious	.04	.06	.05	.12	.05	.21	.41
11. Daydreams	.01	.05	.03	.02	.03	.18	.20
12. Sullen	0	.03	.01	.03	.11	.35	.26
13. Cries	.01	.08	.04	.06	.49	.33	0
14. Disturbs	0	.02	0	.04	0	.09	.01
15. Quarrelsome	.01	.03	.02	.06	.07	.13	.10
16. Moods	.02	.08	0	.01	.23	.32	.17
17. Acts smart	.02	.01	.02	.02	.17	.26	.12
18. Destructive	.02	.02	0	.05	.04	.15	.06
19. Steals	0	.09	.01	.05	.18	.15	.16
20. Lies	0	.13	.01	.02	.15	.07	.20
21. Temper	.03	.13	.01	.07	.30	.27	.01
22. Isolates	.02	0	.05	.10	.02	.18	.46
23. Unaccepted	.03	.15	.07	.07	.31	.09	.21
24. Easily led	.02	0	.04	0	.01	.02	.09
25. No fair play	.01	.03	0	.04	.15	.07	.02
26. Leadership	.01	.04	.03	.04	.04	.03	0
27. Opposite sex	.03	.21	.05	.06	.43	.07	.17
28. Same sex	.02	.19	.05	.07	.40	.04	.18
29. Teases	.01	.02	.03	.07	.16	.04	.02
30. Submissive	.01	.01	.01	.01	.02	.33	.37
31. Defiant	.03	.07	.03	.07	.18	.05	.10
32. Impudent	.02	.03	.01	0	.10	.12	.08
33. Shy	.01	.02	.02	.04	.01	0	.12
34. Fearful	.01	.04	.02	.07	0	0	.07
35. Excessive	.03	.03	.02	.12	.04	.17	.33
36. Stubborn	.02	.04	.01	0	.07	.11	.09
37. Anxious	.01	.01	0	.05	.03	.60	.67
38. Uncooperative	0	.01	0	.03	.07	.18	.21
39. Attendance	.01	.04	.01	0	.10	.02	.02
Number of unstable items	2	18	10	23	30	31	31

* Measure of the difference between test-retest $\sqrt{R.C.}$ is greater than .03

TABLE 14.6

TEST-RETEST RELIABILITY OF UNROTATED FACTORS BASED ON ITEMS GENERALLY USED TO INTERPRET THE FACTORS

		ITEMS																																						No. of items appearing at least once from test to retest	No. of items not appearing in both ratings
FACTORS		1	2	3	4	5	6	7	8	9	10	11	12	13	14	15	16	17	18	19	20	21	22	23	24	25	26	27	28	29	30	31	32	33	34	35	36	37	38	39		
F-1	T	*	*	*		*	*	*	*				*		*	*	*		*		*	*				*		*	*	*		*	*			*	*				23	1
	R	*	*	*		*	*	*	*				*		*	*	*	*	*		*	*				*		*	*	*		*	*			*	*					
F-2	T				*						*	*		*									*	*	*		*							*	*						10	2
	R				*						*	*											*		*		*							*	*							
F-3	T	*		*				*	*	*	*		*	*	*		*					*			*		*			*								*			21	10
	R	*				*	*	*	*		*	*	*		*		*		*	*	*	*			*		*											*				
F-4	T	*	*	*		*	*			*								*	*	*	*			*		*		*	*							*		*			17	9
	R			*						*								*		*	*					*					*					*		*				
F-5	T								*			*	*			*	*				*		*		*		*	*		*	*				*		*	*		21	16
	R							*	*					*		*				*				*				*	*	*		*			*							
F-6	T	*	*			*			*			*							*	*			*								*			*	*	*				*	22	18
	R		*								*		*	*			*			*	*					*	*				*					*		*	*			
F-7	T		*	*				*	*		*		*	*						*	*		*					*					*			*		*			27	24
	R				*	*	*			*		*		*								*	*	*	*						*			*	*			*	*	*		

* – the loading on this factor is in absolute value $\geq \sqrt{\frac{\text{contribution of factor}}{39}}$

the test–retest reliability of a factor unpredictably changes. Again, the mathematical procedures applied to the data creates a test–retest instability.

TABLE 14.7

TEST-RETEST RELIABILITY OF ROTATED FACTORS BASED ON ITEMS GENERALLY USED TO INTERPRET THE FACTORS

		ITEMS																																						No. of items appearing at least once from test to retest	No. of items not appearing in both ratings
FACTORS		1	2	3	4	5	6	7	8	9	10	11	12	13	14	15	16	17	18	19	20	21	22	23	24	25	26	27	28	29	30	31	32	33	34	35	36	37	38	39		
F-1	T	*	*			*	*	*							*	*		*												*		*	*			*					15	4
	R	*	*	*		*	*	*							*	*													*	*		*	*			*	*					
F-2	T												*			*			*	*	*	*		*		*		*	*	*		*	*				*		*		16	7
	R															*	*		*	*	*	*				*							*				*		*			
F-3	T				*						*	*											*		*		*				*			*	*						10	2
	R				*					*	*												*		*		*				*			*	*							
F-4	T			*	*			*	*			*											*	*			*				*					*			*	*	12	1
	R				*			*	*			*											*	*			*				*					*			*	*		
F-5	T			*						*			*	*		*	*			*	*	*															*				20	18
	R		*								*		*			*		*	*					*		*		*	*	*		*										
F-6	T			*						*								*													*					*		*			13	11
	R			*						*	*		*	*			*					*											*				*					
F-7	T										*	*	*				*	*		*	*		*	*				*	*			*	*				*				20	19
	R			*						*								*													*					*		*	*			

* – the loading on this factor is in absolute value $\geq \sqrt{\frac{\text{contribution of factor}}{39}}$

TABLE 14.8

TEST-RETEST RELIABILITY OF FACTOR I BASED ON ITEMS GENERALLY USED TO INTERPRET THE FACTOR

AFTER ROTATION OF K = 3, 4, 5, 6, 7 FACTORS

FACTORS	ITEMS																																							No. of items appearing at least once from test to retest	No. of items not appearing in both ratings
	1	2	3	4	5	6	7	8	9	10	11	12	13	14	15	16	17	18	19	20	21	22	23	24	25	26	27	28	29	30	31	32	33	34	35	36	37	38	39		
K − 3 T	*	*	*	*	*	*	*					*		*	*	*		*		*	*				*		*	*	*		*	*			*	*				26	13
R			*									*			*	*	*	*	*	*	*		*		*		*	*			*	*				*					
K − 4 T	*	*	*		*	*	*	*						*	*														*		*	*			*					14	3
R	*	*			*	*	*	*						*	*														*		*				*	*					
K − 5 T	*	*	*		*	*	*	*						*	*														*		*				*					19	11
R	*	*			*	*								*	*		*	*							*		*	*	*		*	*				*					
K − 6 T	*	*	*		*	*	*	*						*	*														*		*				*					21	12
R	*	*			*	*						*		*	*		*	*					*		*		*	*	*		*	*				*					
K − 7 T	*	*			*	*	*							*	*		*												*		*	*			*					15	4
R	*	*	*		*	*	*							*	*													*	*		*	*			*	*					

* — the "loading" in absolue value $> \sqrt{\frac{\text{contribution of factor}}{39}}$

(c) Thirdly, we calculated the correlation coefficients between the loadings of the unrotated factors from test to retest and the results are given in Table 14.8. If one accepts the correlation coefficient as the appropriate measure of T–R reliability, then, depending on the cut-points usually chosen for this category of data, one would accept the first four or five factors to be T–R reliable. Considering what has been found by the previous two methods, this raises an interesting question: What is the best method to assess the T–R reliability of factors? Obviously, the answer to that question depends on which aspects of the reliability of a factor are most important to a specific research question. The correlation coefficient method provides a good T–R reliability of scores pertaining to a given set of questions; one accepts the reliability even though there are questions within the set that are T–R unreliable. For this reason, it follows that if one is interested in ideas represented by few items in the questionnaire (e.g., inattention or poor coordination), asking himself in which general factors these more fine-grained ideas will appear, then the correlation coefficient method is clearly not the most suitable method to assess the T–R reliability of a factor. For this kind of question, one has to use a method that assesses the T–R reliability for every question according to some defined criteria.

Interpretation of the Factors

If, before interpreting a factor, we want to make sure that it is a reliable factor and that it explains a significant proportion of the variance, then the

TABLE 14.9 *Factor I (Test—without rotation)*

Items		Loading on F-1
1.	Fidgeting (b)	.73
2.	Hums (b)	.67
3.	Demands must be met immediately; gets frustrated (a, b)	.64
5.	Restless (b)	.69
6.	Excitable, impulsive (b)	.75
7.	Inattentive; distractable (c)	.65
8.	Short attention span (c)	.57
12.	Sullen or sulky (a)	.67
14.	Disturbs other children (a)	.77
15.	Quarrelsome (a)	.81
16.	Mood changes quickly (a)	.70
18.	Destructive (a)	.65
20.	Lies (a)	.61
21.	Temper outbursts (a)	.64
25.	No sense of fair play (a)	.69
27.	Does not get along with opposite sex (a)	.65
28.	Does not get along with same sex (a)	.71
29.	Teases other children or interferes with their activities (a, b)	.77
31.	Defiant (a)	.73
32.	Impudent (a)	.66
35.	Excessive	.67
36.	Stubborn	.72
N = 22		Cut point = $\sqrt{\frac{\lambda}{39}}$ = .56

Main idea: *Outward type of behavior*:
Conduct Disorder (a) Inattention (c)
Hyperactivity (b)

most important factors to interpret, according to our study, are F-1 and F-2 of the unrotated methods.

The first factor (Table 14.9) clearly identifies an outward type of behavior, more precisely examplified by the ideas of conduct disorder,

TABLE 14.10 *Factor II (Test—without rotation)*

Items		Loading on F-2
4.	Coordination poor (c)	.55
10.	Serious or sad (b)	.50
11.	Daydreams	.52
13.	Cries	.33
22.	Isolates himself from other children (a)	.60
23.	Appears to be unaccepted by group	.34
24.	Appears to be easily led (a)	.71
26.	Appears to lack leadership (a)	.73
33.	Shy (b)	.74
34.	Fearful (b)	.73
N = 10		Cut point = $\sqrt{\frac{\lambda}{39}}$ = .33

Main idea: *Inward type of behavior*:
Passivity (a) Coordination (c)
Inhibition (b)

TABLE 14.11 *Comparison between Trites' first factor and our Factor I obtained after rotation of K = 3...7 factors at test and retest*

	Items	K = 6	K = 3		K = 4		K = 5		K = 6		K = 7	
		Trites*	T	R	T	R	T	R	T	R	T	R
1.	Fidgeting (b)	×	×		×	×	×	×	×	×	×	×
2.	Hums (b)	×	×		×	×	×	×	×	×	×	×
3.	Demands (a, b)	×	×	×	×		×		×			×
4.	Coordination	+	×									
5.	Restless (b)	×	×		×	×	×	×	×	×	×	×
6.	Excitable (b)	×	×		×	×	×	×	×	×	×	×
7.	Inattentive (c)	×	×		×	×	×		×		×	×
8.	Short span (c)	×			×	×	×		×			
9.	Sensitive											
10.	Serious											
11.	Daydreams	+										
12.	Sullen (a)		×	×						×		
13.	Cries											
14.	Disturbs (a, b)	×		×	×	×	×	×	×	×	×	×
15.	Quarrelsome (a)	+	×	×	×	×	×	×	×	×	×	×
16.	Moods (a)		×	×								
17.	Acts smart (a)	+		×				×		×	×	
18.	Destructive (a)		×	×				×		×		
19.	Steals (a)			×								
20.	Lies (a)		×	×								
21.	Temper (a)		×	×								
22.	Isolates											
23.	Unaccepted			×						×		
24.	Easily led	+										
25.	No fair play (a)		×	×				×		×		
26.	Leadership											
27.	Opposite sex (a)		×	×				×		×		×
28.	Same sex (a)		×	×				×		×		
29.	Teases (a, b)	×		×	×	×	×	×	×	×	×	×
30.	Submissive											
31.	Defiant (a)		×	×	×	×	×	×	×	×	×	×
32.	Impudent (a)	+	×	×	×			×		×	×	×
33.	Shy											
34.	Fearful											
35.	Excessive (a, b)	+		×	×	×	×		×		×	×
36.	Stubborn (a)		×	×	×			×		×		×
37.	Anxious											
38.	Uncooperative	+										
39.	Attendance											

$\times > \sqrt{\dfrac{\text{contribution of factor}}{39}}$

$+ < \sqrt{\dfrac{\text{contribution of factor}}{39}}$

Conduct Disorder (a)
Hyperactivity (b)
Inattention (c)

*From Trites, R. L., *et al.*, 1982.

hyperactivity and inattention. Our second reliable factor is important to inward types of behavior, that is, passivity and inhibition (Table 14.10).

As can be seen, hyperactivity does not emerge as an independent factor in our data. Hyperactivity was found to be associated to conduct disorder.

This fact has been described elsewhere for other questionnaires and by Kupietz (1974) for the CTQ. It has recently been argued by Trites (1982) that a primary hyperactivity factor was not obtained in previous studies of the CTQ because large enough nonclinical populations were not used. The present study bears on what we might call a large nonclinical sample and whether or not our first factor, obtained through the varimax procedure, supports Trites' statement depends either on the number of factors retained for the rotation or whether we choose the factors obtained at the test or at the retest. Table 14.11 illustrates that, because of the instability of the rotated factors, one can choose factors that will have practically the same loadings found by Trites (K = 4 at retest), or factors that will have different loadings (K = 6 retest or K = 3 retest).

CONCLUSIONS

We found 37 of 39 test–retest questions reliable for the Conners Teacher Questionnaire. Even though the great majority of the questions are test–retest reliable, only two unrotated factors (the first two) were found to be consistently test–retest reliable.

The varimax rotation unpredictably introduced test–retest unreliability into the structure and, consequently, caution is indicated for the clinical interpretation of rotated factors. The two factors found to be reliable describe: (a) an outward type of behavior (conduct, hyperactivity and inattention); and (b) an inward type of behavior (passivity, inhibition, to which is associated poor coordination).

GENERAL DISCUSSION

Dr. Swanson: You developed your own unique method to (a) make a judgment about the size of a significant factor loading and (b) compare factors obtained by one analysis with those obtained from another. Such a method leads you to conclude that the unrotated factors, which are reliable, are a very limited number, even more limited than the rotated factors. While your method may have considerable promise, at this point it needs to be compared with other more widely accepted methods of determining whether factors from one analysis are comparable to those from another. The value in comparing your method with the value comparisons with standard methods is probably far beyond what it says about the Conners.

Dr. Coté: If the correlation coefficient computed is something like 0.6, 0.7, 0.8, 0.4, I could say: "I've got high correlation coefficients and you might say this is not a high correlation coefficient." With this new method, I can adjust it. I check all values instead of having one number to assess the entire array of loadings.

Dr. Swanson: If 3 factors are rotated you get a pattern different from that when 5 factors or 6 factors are rotated. Thus, the choice and number of factors allowed affects their test–retest reliability. As there are an infinite number of rotations, you are in an indeterminant system. In factor analysis, an unrotated analysis is better used.

Dr. Quay: Simple structure was the best you could get and the Varimax program was the best mathematical approximation to simple structure. There are really two reasons a factor analysis is done from my point of view. First, if you want to discover the underlying structure of a data domain, then there are choices you want to make. Second, factor analysis is used to construct a measuring instrument. Then your criteria for constructing factor scales should be to maximize the reliability of the scale, to minimize its intercorrelation with other scales, and to maximize its correlation with some external criteria. The Varimax is the best approximation we have to simple structure. It maximizes factor variance by trying to make the loading as close to 0 or 1 as is possible, which is what is wanted for simple structure. You want as many zero loadings and as many 1 loadings as possible within the mathematical constraints of the rotation, preserving the angle between factors and the communality of the items.

Dr. Hunt: If you sampled 100 ADD children, each from three distinct clinical subtypes, one group high in levels of aggression, another group selected for co-existent conduct disorder, and a third group of ADD children who were unusually hyperactive, would the differences in the clinical characteristics of the children be likely to produce factors different from the Varimax rotation of scores on behavior ratings?

Dr. Thivierge: With populations that have different characteristics the factors you are going to obtain are obviously important in differentiating them.

Dr. Hunt: Then the factors you obtain through this analysis of the scale will depend on the clinical characteristics of the population sampled and may be very different from the factors obtained in another population. Can you utilize the factors derived from one population to scale or quantify the behavior of another population, or should you first repeat the rotational analysis to see if the same facts emerge?

Dr. Thivierge: The only population we can compare ours to is Dr. Trites' population because it bears on a nonclinical population like ours. Most other studies have been done on clinical populations.

Dr. Hunt: How much can one infer from the factors you derived from normal children when applying this scale to a group of ADD children?

Dr. Thivierge: The only point we are making in this respect is that when we do Principal Component Analysis, we check the reliability of the factors we obtain. What's the use of having, for instance, a very simple group of questions if this group turns out to be a nonreliable structure? We have some evidence that some instability is being created by the Varimax rotation.

Dr. Swanson: If we try to use the Conners questionnaire and the factors on the Conners to subgroup children, are we dealing with a reliable instrument so that noise is not such that we do not have noise introduced into the subgroup of patients?

Dr. Thivierge: Before we use the factors in one population, we have to factor analyze the questionnaire. One can practically choose any grouping of questions within the Conners and find a good test/retest reliability on the scores. Why? Because the questions are reliable. So the Principal Component Analysis gives a particular grouping of questions to which you attach a certain meaning, otherwise you wouldn't do it. The grouping is the important factor.

Dr. Swanson: In talking about test–retest reliability of factors, I've always thought that factors were used to subgroup children. If the Conners' factor analysis, where there were separate factors, is used and the score applied to subgroup children very low on conduct disorder and very high on hyperactivity, are we dealing with something that is unreliable and introducing noise into the subgroupings?

Dr. Thivierge: I don't think you are dealing with something unreliable because the questions are reliable. By Principal Component Analysis we obtain a set of questions that most differentiate our children but this conclusion does not necessarily apply to your population. You have to do your own factor analysis on your population to attach meaning to the factor you obtained. This is particularly true when one gives importance to ideas that are being represented by a very limited number of questions.

Dr. Swanson: So you do your own normative study to get local factors before you analyze your data. No one does that.

Dr. Thivierge: Kupietz (1974) has said that everyone should be doing it and I agree with him.

REFERENCES

Capéraà P, Côté R, Thivierge J: Hyperactivity: Comment on Trites' Article. Journal of Child Psychology and Psychiatry 1985; 26:485–486.

ECDEU: Assessment Manual for Psychopharmacology. US Department of Health Education and Welfare, NIMH, 1976.

Klotz JH: Testing a linear constraint for multinomial frequencies and disease screenery. The Annals of Statistics 1978; 6:904–1090.

Kupietz S, Botti E: Behavior measurement in pediatric psychopharmacology. Am J Psychiat 1974; 131:106.

Magnusson D: Test Theory. Reading Mass, Addison Wesley, 1967, p 59.

Trites RL, Blouin AGA, Laprade K: Factor analysis of the Conners teacher rating scale based on a large normative sample. J Consult Clin Psychol 1982; 50:615–623.

15

Controlled Prospective Fifteen Year Follow-up of Hyperactives as Adults Non-medical Drug and Alcohol Use and Antisocial Behavior*

LILY HECHTMAN AND GABRIELLE WEISS

EDITOR'S SYNOPSIS

An initial cohort of 104 hyperactive children, without organic brain damage, psychosis or mental retardation, participated in acute drug studies with amphetamines and phenothiazines for several weeks although they received no sustained stimulant treatment. Of these subjects, initially age 6–12 years, 91 were followed through adolescence and 75 of the 91 into young adulthood, 17–24 years (mean: 19). Sixty-one subjects (81% of the 10-year follow-up) were studied after 15 years.

In the 5-year follow-up study of adolescents, a matched control group was selected of volunteers among high school classmates of the hyperactive subjects. Of 45 controls at the 10-year follow-up, 41 (91%) participated in the 15-year evaluation that included two self-rating scales; Symptom Check List–90 (SCL–90) and the California Psychological Inventory (CPI). Results showed that the controls showed a trend ($p < 0.06$) to have a slightly higher mean IQ than hyperactive (108 vs. 104). No significant differences between controls and hyperactives were found in the use of alcohol and non-medical drugs, although there was a trend for more hyperactives to be involved in selling (13 vs. 3) ($p < 0.09$). The findings on alcohol and drug use were confirmed with a subgroup (37 controls, 51 hyperactives) who agreed to do the SADS.

In the last three years of the study, more hyperactive subjects tended to be involved in court appearances than controls (11 vs. 2) ($p < 0.09$). The total number of court appearances was also higher for the hyperactives (24 vs. 2) ($p < 0.07$).

More hyperactive subjects tended to have problems with physical aggression when compared to controls (12 vs. 1) ($p < 0.07$). A global assessment scale revealed that for antisocial behavior the numbers of hyperactives vs. controls did not differ significantly. However, the severity of antisocial behavior was much greater in the hyperactive group ($p < 0.01$).

Using a purely clinical definition, one of 41 controls and 14 of 61 hyperactives were judged to be antisocial ($p < 0.01$). Using strict SADS criteria, none of the controls and one hyperactive had antisocial personality disorder (ASPD). Using a modified SADS without questions pertinent to DSM-III, one control and 14 hyperactives received a diagnosis of ASPD ($p < 0.01$). DSM-III criteria yielded the same numbers.

Regrettably Chapter 15 had to be replaced by this editor's synopsis due to publication demands and because this material appears in a more comprehensive form in Weiss G, Hechtman LT: Hyperactive Children Grown Up: Empirical Findings and Theoretical Considerations. New York: The Guilford Press, 1986. Copies of the chapter may be obtained from Lily T. Hechtman, M.D., Department of Psychiatry, The Montreal Children's Hospital, 2300 Tupper Street, Montreal, Quebec H3H 1P3, Canada.

16

The Behavioral Reward and Inhibition System in Childhood Behavior Disorder

HERBERT C. QUAY

In a series of conceptual and empirical papers, Jeffrey A. Gray has set forth a theory of brain function that underlies the various paradigms of learning, already familiar to psychologists (for recent summaries, see Gray, 1972a, 1972b, 1973, 1979, 1982). In Gray's framework, increases in responding brought about by positive reinforcement and by both active avoidance and escape paradigms are under control of a reward system (REW). This system is sensitive to signals of reward ("hope") and of nonpunishment ("relief"). On the other hand, reduced responding in passive avoidance and extinction is controlled by a behavioral inhibition system (BIS), sensitive to signals of impending punishment (PUN) ("fear" in passive avoidance) and frustrative nonreward (FNR) ("frustration" in extinction).

For Gray, anxiety is activity in the BIS cued by conditioned stimuli that signal fear or frustration (see Gray, 1979). He reaches this conclusion by examining the effects of antianxiety drugs (e.g., alcohol, barbiturates, benzodiazepines) that have been shown to impair both passive avoidance and to increase resistance to extinction; behaviors under the control of the BIS. Furthermore, the antianxiety drugs do not impair behavior under the control of the REW, so that their effects are selective on the BIS.

Gray has also proposed anatomic loci for these two systems. His reward system corresponds to those responsible for the rewarding effects of electric self-stimulation (see Olds and Fobes, 1981 for a review). These pathways are catecholaminergic. The locus of the BIS is in the lateral and medial septal areas and in the connections of the areas to the hippocampus; the Septohippocampal System. According to Gray the BIS is noradrenergic (see Gray, 1979).

Gray has also speculated on the relationship of these two (actually three, including the fight/flight system) systems to psychopathology. (A third system, flight-fight, reacts to unconditioned punishing stimuli by mediating withdrawal or aggression depending upon the environmental circumstances. On the other hand, predatory aggression is under the control of REW.) The anxious/depressive-type disorders appear to be related to excessive sensitivity to signals of PUN and FNR mediated by the BIS. Externalizing disorders, especially psychopathy, may reflect an underactive BIS, or an overactive REW, or perhaps the dominance of the latter over the former.

My purpose is to attempt to place three broad-band childhood disorders—Attention Deficit Disorder with Hyperactivity (ADDH), Conduct Disorder (CD), and Anxiety-Withdrawal Disorder (AW)—within Gray's REW and BIS model. I will then propose a number of investigations, utilizing both learning paradigms and psychophysiologic measures to test those proposed relationships.

ADDH: OVERACTIVE REW OR UNDERACTIVE BIS?

Is the behavior of the ADDH child determined by an oversusceptible REW or by an underactive BIS? We know that the ADDH child does poorly in situations requiring the withholding of responses. For example, he makes errors of commission in continuous performance tasks and is unable to inhibit responding on a DRL schedule (Gordon 1979). At the same time, delivery of reward during learning has been reported to disrupt performance. However, this effect has been interpreted as possibly due to an inability to inhibit responses to the rewards themselves (see Douglas and Peters, 1979 for a review).

If REW is already hypersensitive, then REW agonists should be further disruptive. However, we know that:

1. Dextroamphetamine facilitates self-stimulation in the medial forebrain bundle, a noradrenergic tract (Olds and Fobes, 1981). Thus, dextroamphetamine enhances the activity of the REW.
2. The BIS, activated through the dorsal ascending noradrenergic bundle, should respond to dextroamphetamine.
3. Behaviorally, dextroamphetamine improves inhibitory behavior (passive avoidance) in ADDH.
4. While dextroamphetamine enhances both reward and inhibitory systems, the behavioral effect suggests that there must be relatively greater enhancement of the BIS function to bring it into balance with the REW.
5. Conversely, antianxiety drugs, which adversely affect only the BIS, should make ADDH children worse, which they seem to do.

We may note in passing, that ADDH cases which are nonresponsive to d-amphetamine may be cases whose REW is overactive so that any increment in the BIS function is offset by an increment in heightened sensitivity to reward.

The preponderance of evidence, both behavioral and pharmacologic, suggests a deficient BIS as being implicated in the pathogenesis of ADDH.

To test this hypothesis, we may make use of various learning processes that Gray has argued are related to the BIS:

Extinction

1. Extinction is controlled by the BIS, which serves to extinguish responding after nonreward (FNR).
2. Antianxiety drugs *increase* resistance to extinction, by decreasing the BIS.
3. An underactive BIS should result in higher resistance to extinction (reduced effects of FNR).

Therefore, ADDH children should show higher resistance to extinction.

Fixed Interval (FI), Fixed Ratio (FR), and Differential Reinforcement of Low Rate (DRL) Schedules of Reinforcement

1. FI, FR and FRL schedules include an event that signals, for some period of time, nonreinforcement, an event that serves as a conditioned frustrative stimulus.
2. Signals of FNR activate the BIS.
3. An underactive BIS should result in increased rates of responding.
4. Antianxiety drugs that antogonize the BIS increase rates of responding under these schedules.

Thus, if ADDH children are deficient in the BIS, they should show higher rates of responding under FI, FR, and DRL schedules. (This has been already demonstrated by Gordon, 1979).

The Partial Reinforcement Extinction Effect

1. Partial reinforcement (PRF) increases resistance to extinction, since tolerance develops for FNR.
2. The extinction effect of partial reinforcement (PREE) is under control of the BIS, which reacts to the FNR.
3. Antianxiety drugs attenuate the effects of PREE by antogonizing the BIS.
4. Underfunctioning of the BIS should attentuate PREE.

Thus, ADDH children show less PREE.

Behavioral Contrast and Peak Shift

1. Both behavioral contrast and peak shift are due to consequences of effects of FNR associated with a negative stimulus.
2. Such effects are a function of susceptibility to frustration (controlled by the BIS).
3. An underfunctioning BIS should result in less susceptability to FNR and in less contrast and peak shift.

Therefore, ADDH children should show less behavioral contrast and peak shift.

CONDUCT DISORDER: OVERSENSITIVE REW OR AN UNDERACTIVE BIS?

As in the case of ADDH, severe CD children (and adult psychopaths) are known to be deficient in withholding responses. It is also known that:

1. Amphetamine, a REW and BIS agonist, improves passive avoidance but does not improve conduct disordered behavior (Campbell *et al.*, 1982).
2. Thus, a drug that facilitates both REW and the BIS does not improve CD.
3. However, both propanolol and haloperidol antagonize REW as they reduce brain self-stimulation and antagonize DA (and NE). There is at least suggestive evidence that catecholamine antagonists decrease CD behavior, although sedation effects are possible here (Campbell *et al.*, 1982).

Thus, CD seems most related to oversensitivity to reward.

Anxiety-Withdrawal Disorder: An Excess of BIS

The internalizing, anxiety-type disorders are the prototype for an overactive BIS. Anxiety facilitates passive avoidance and increases resistance to extinction. The antianxiety drugs antagonize the BIS and serve to "disinhibit" the behavior of the anxiety neurotic.

DIFFERENTIAL PERFORMANCE OF THE THREE DISORDERS IN INSTRUMENTAL LEARNING

Is it now possible to make some differential predictions about the performance of all three groups with respect to the conditions of learning?

As noted, Gray asserts that reward learning, active avoidance, and escape learning are controlled by REW, while passive avoidance and extinction are controlled by the BIS. Thus, some differences would be

TABLE 16.1

Hypothesized Relative Performance of the Three Groups in Five Learning Paradigms

	Reward			Punish	
	Reward (Respond)	Avoid (Respond)	Escape (Respond)	Passive Avoid (Inhibit)	Rapidity of Extinction (Inhibit)
ADDH	+	+	+	--	--
CD	++	++	++	-	-
AW	-	-	-	++	++
Normal (No)	+	+	+	+	+

Reward:	CD > ADDH = No > AW
Avoidance:	CD > ADDH = No > AW
Escape:	CD > ADDH = No > AW
Passive Avoidance:	AW > No > CD > ADDH
Rapidity of Extinction:	AW > No > CD > ADDH

ADDH:	REW > PUN
CD:	REW > PUN
AW:	PUN > REW
No:	REW = PUN

expected in performance in these forms of instrumental learning among the three groups. These hypothesized differences are set out in Table 16.1.

The CD group should outperform the other two groups in all three conditions involving REW, with the ADDHs and normals "tied" for second. Under the BIS mediated conditions, the AW group should outperform all others, with the ADDH group least successful. In passing, it is noted that while many studies of learning in all three groups have been done, no study has compared all three groups plus normals under all five conditions, with predictions made, *a priori*, on the basis of Gray's theory.

Generalization

Gray (Nicholson and Gray, 1972; Gray, 1972a) has suggested that "the tendency to generalize can only reflect the activity of the "reward mechanism" (Nicholson and Gray, 1972; p 60). Furthermore, generalization should increase with increasing "neuroticism" *and* extroversion.

If our analysis of ADDH, CD and AW are correct, then the greatest generalization would be expected in the CD group (since CD subjects are, in Eysenck-Gray terminology, "extroverted neurotics"). The next greatest generalization should be among ADDH children, since the former are highly neurotic but not extraverted, while the latter, in our opinion, are extroverted but not anxious. Normal controls should show the least generalization.

The role played by the BIS in generalization if any, is not specified by Gray.

ADDH and the Measurement of Autonomic Nervous System (ANS) Variables

To date, measurements of autonomic function have not been the "royal road" to understanding ADDH. Results have been contradictory regarding phasic arousal and there has been no consistent difference in tonic levels between ADD children and normal controls. Even when the influences of CD and anxiety have been looked at separately, results have not been consistent (e.g., Delameter and Lahey, 1982; Zweben *et al.*, unpublished data).

Recent theorizing by Fowles (1983), however, has opened the possibility of a less "shotgun" approach to ANS measurement to elucidate nervous system function in ADDH, CD, and AW. Fowles maintains that *heart rate* (HR) does *not* index anxiety (the BIS) but rather is more closely linked to appetitive motivation (the REW). On the other hand, electrodermal activity is associated with inhibition and anxiety (the BIS). If these two measures do, in fact, differentially index Gray's two systems, then predictions can be made on the basis of subject variables interacting with task variables. We note here that while Zweben *et al.* (unpublished data) did not find differences in GSR responsivity as a function of type of disorder, they found negative correlations between errors of commission on a brief continuous performance task and measure of GSR responsivity across all subjects. This would, of course, suggest a negative relationship between BIS function and the Galvanic skin response (GSR) responsivity as predicted by Fowles (1983).

Table 16.2 outlines one possible attack on the investigation of differences in functioning in the two systems in ADDH, CD, and AW, compared to normals.

Under conditions of incentive motivation, which bring REW into play, HR changes should be greater in CD children, next greater and equal in normals and ADDH children, and least in AW. If activation of the BIS

TABLE 16.2

Hypothesized Heart Rate and GSR Responsivity in the Four Groups Under Reward and Inhibition Conditions

	Incentive Conditions				Passive Avoidance Conditions			
	Normal	ADD	CD	AW	Normal	ADD	CD	AW
HR	++	++	+++	+	0	0	0	0
GSR	0	0	0	0	+	0	+	++

Incentive HR: CD > ADD = Normal = AW

Incentive GSR: CD = ADD = Normal = AW

Incentive: HR > GSR (how to tell?)

Passive Avoidance HR: CD = ADD = Normal = AW

Passive Avoidance GSR: AW > Normal > CD > ADD

Passive Avoidance: GSR > HR (how to tell?)

can be avoided, there should be minimal and equal GSR reactivity in all groups.

In a passive avoidance situation, the BIS is energized so that the greatest GSR changes would appear in the AW group; the next greater in CD and normals (equally); and the least in the ADDH group.

Heart Rate and Generalization

Finally, we propose that if generalization is a measure of individual susceptability to reward and HR relates to the REW then, at least under incentive conditions, there should be a positive correlation between HR during learning and generalization following learning in all four groups.

Work in all of these areas is now getting underway. As suggested in the previous volume of this series (Quay, 1984), careful subject selection is imperative if we are to make progress. We hope we are successful in this, as well as in surmounting a host of other methodolgic problems.

GENERAL DISCUSSION

Dr. Simeon: What is the skin conductance response in schizophrenics?

Dr. Quay: I can't comment on skin conductance with respect to schizophrenia but the one consistent autonomic system finding in psychopaths is lower levels of electrodermal arousability.

Dr. Sergeant: In the high-risk study for schizophrenia, there was low tonic skin conductance with low phasic activity. There was a faster recovery rate on the high risk for schizophrenic children versus the normal recovery rate in the psychopath group.

Dr. Klorman: That sample had an excess of psychopathic fathers, which make it an idiosyncratic sample of children with schizophrenic mothers (Kirkeguard-Sorensen and Mednick, 1975).

Dr. Satterfield: Several studies have compared ADDH and normal children and consistently found that the autonomic response is a low skin conductance response.

Dr. Quay: That agrees with the theory that ADDH children have an underactive behavioral inhibition system (BIS).

Dr. Hunt: Your discussion provides a broader behavioral and conceptual model, which parallels our neurochemical observations. Your data are also congruent with the findings of Mason and Iverson (1982) regarding the dorsal bundle extinction effect. The dorsal noradrenergic tract (bundle), emanating from the locus coeruleus, was obliterated chemically or electrically in rats prior to continuously re-enforced acquisition learning. Rate of learning did not change but after re-enforcement was discontinued, the rats exhibited an extended extinction phase, suggesting they may have been internally distracted—they were learning under conditions analogous to intermittent enforcement, following which extinction is typically prolonged. You may have provided the framework for understanding some of the effects of clonidine, because clinically it appears that the drug increases inhibition, which may be what the parents described as an increase in frustration tolerance.

Dr. Sergeant: Have you observed baseline habituation?

Dr. Quay: These measures are not totally independent of one another, so that baseline skin conductance response frequency, habituation in skin frequency, active task frequency and active task response magnitude are interrelated.

Dr. Sergeant: The lower the skin conductance, apparently the higher your commission error rate. Is a low commission rate the same kind of cognitive process as passive avoidance?

Dr. Quay: Withholding the response to the incorrect stimulus is a passive avoidance task.

Dr. Sergeant: What was the speed of errors of commission? On the same model, you would be predicting that there would be fast errors of commission. If this is correct then the speed of processing would predictably be faster for errors of commission than for correct hits, because the latter reflect true processing whereas the former, or fast guesses, reflect loss of inhibitory control.

Dr. Quay: Errors of commission have shorter latencies.

Dr. Simeon: What type of anxiety are you talking about—the tendency for worries, phobias, concerns or the very inhibited, shy, withdrawn, nervous child. Other types of anxiety, like panic states and school phobia respond to antidepressants and not to antianxiety drugs.

Dr. Quay: Gray is talking about the anxiety responsive to antianxiety drugs and has shown that the BIS can effectively be destroyed. There will be no effect on reward learning, passive avoidance learning will be seriously impaired, and there will be increased resistance to extinction.

Dr. Ferguson: In the late '70s, people became more careful about selecting their autonomic research groups. Measures, which tend to show differences, are in fact skin potential measures. Although there are quite a few heart rate differences, good psychophysiologists, (e.g. Zahn *et al.*, 1975), did not find consistent differences in habituation. How do you reconcile your findings with those of the psychophysiologists of long-standing reputation?

Dr. Quay: Your analysis is counter to the notion that ADD is an inhibition disorder; ADD children would be expected to show less rapid extinction. Many studies showing a difference in skin potentials report fewer spontaneous skin responses in hyperactive groups, not more. If there is a failure in the inhibition system, more frequent spontaneous responses would be expected.

Dr. Ferguson: I predict fewer spontaneous responses, because that would indicate less activity in the inhibition system, as suggested by these tonic and phasic measures.

Dr. Quay: If the inhibition system is less active, the excitatory system would be expected to stimulate responses more frequently, as they are less supressed by the inhibition system. I have simply tried to test the extreme hypothesis first.

Dr. Pelham: The discussion suggests that conduct disorder behaviors do not respond to stimulant medication. Most of the data I have seen suggest that these behaviors improve tremendously.

Dr. Satterfield: We are looking at specific target conduct disorder behaviors, like fighting and agressivity, in terms of response to stimulant drugs. Our group showed a definite, significant response to stimulant medication.

Dr. Klorman: I showed a decrease on Loney's measure of aggression in the double-blind trial in Chapter 4 of this volume. Regarding autonomic measures, perhaps a sharper design would more clearly test the implications of your formulation. In a continuous performance test, the rate of stimulus presentation is typically very frequent, every few seconds, a boring situation that challenges the subject. Because of the latency in autonomic response, the response to a particular stimulus cannot be identified because they are so frequent. A rate of every 10 seconds or longer is required. I would suggest a study design utilizing a format that permits such differentiation. Studies in the literature on ADD used formats that permit the detection of individual stimuli in reaction time tasks. Stroufe's, Porges' or Zahn's work (Stroufe *et al.*, 1973; Porges *et al.*, 1975; Zahn *et al.*, 1975) clearly show smaller responses to attention evoked stimuli. They may not have differentiated between positive and negative stimuli.

Dr. Sergeant: A study of evoked responses showed the magnitude of the P300 component was related to the value of the stimulus, causing me to think that the evoked response was a window to the reward system.

Dr. Klorman: Not specifically to the target and nontarget. You may predict differences as a function of a positive or negative stimulus, that the autonomic measure was heart rate or skin conductance and whether it was reward or not.

Dr. Swanson: Gray's work on the partial reinforcement extinction effect and response in the presence of frustration led me to think that the ADD group really fits the theory, but the conduct disordered group would be more problematic. Why did you choose the conduct disordered group, for your initial test of the theory, rather than ADD groups, which seem to have a deficiency in perseverance? Amsel's early work dealt with frustration leading to perseverance on all sorts of tasks later on, whether it is early experience, personality, or constitutional effects. Perseverance seemed to relate to attention deficit disorder.

REFERENCES

Campbell B, Cohen JL, Small AA: Drugs in aggressive behavior. J Am Acad Child Psychiat 1982; 21:107–117.

Delametee, AM, Lahey BB: Physiological correlates of conduct problems and anxiety in hyperactive and learning-disabled children. J Abnorm Child Psychol 1983; 11:25–100.

Douglas VI, Peters KG: Toward a clearer definition of the attentional deficit of hyperactive children. In Hale and Lewis (eds): Attention and the Development of Cognitive Skills. New York, Plenum Press, 1979.

Fowles DC: Motivational effects on heart rate and electrodermal activity: implications for research in personality and psychopathology. J Res Personal 1983; 17:48–71.

Gordon M: The assessment of impulsivity and mediating behavior in hyperactive and nonhyperactive boys. J Abnorm Child Psychol 1979; 7:317–326.

Gray JA: Learning theory, the conceptual nervous system and personality. In Neblitsin and Gray (eds): Biological Bases of Individual Behavior. New York, Academic Press, 1972a, pp 370–398.

Gray JA: The psychophysiological nature of introversion-extraversion: a modification of Eysenck's theory. In Neblitsin and Gray (eds): Biological Bases of Individual Behavior. New York, Academic Press, 1972b, pp 182–205.

Gray JA: Causal theories of personality and how to test them. In Royce (ed): Multivariate Analysis and Psychological Theory. New York, Academic Press, 1973, pp 409–463.

Gray JA: A neuropsychological theory of anxiety. In Izard (ed): Emotions in Personality and Psychopathology. New York, Plenum Press, 1979, pp 303–335.

Gray JA: The Neuropsychology of Anxiety: an Enquiry into the functions of the Septo-Hippocampal System. New York, Oxford University Press, 1982.

Nicholson JN, Gray JA: Peak shift, behavioural contrast and stimulus generalization as related to personality and development in children. Br J of Psychology, 1972; 63:47–62.

Olds ME, Fobes JC: The central basis of motivation: Intracranial self-stimulation studies. In Rosenzweig and Porter (eds), Annual Review of Psychology. Palto Alto, CA: Annual Reviews, Inc., 1981, pp 523–574.

Porges SW, Walter GF, Korb RJ, Sprague RL: The influences of methylphenidate on heart rate and behavioral measures of attention in hyperactive children. Child Dev. 1975; 46:727–733.

Quay HC: Aggression, conduct disorder, and attention problems. In Bloomingdale (ed): Attention Deficit Disorder: Identification; Course, Treatment Rationale. New York: Spectrum Publications, 1984, pp 33–47.

Stroufe LA, Sonies B, West WP, Wright FS: Anticipatory heart rate deceleration and reaction time in children with and without referral for learning and behavioral disorders. Child Dev 1973; 44:267–273.

Zahn TP, Abate F, Little BC, Wender PH: Minimal brain dysfunction, stimulant drugs, and autonomic nervous system activity. Arch Gen Psychiatr 1975; 32:381–387.

Zweben R, Hammer D, Quay HC: Physiological and behavioral correlates of attentional problems. Conduct problems and anxiety in children. Unpublished paper.

17

Psychosocial Effects on Delinquency Rates in ADD Youths and Control Subjects: An Eight-year Prospective Study

JAMES H. SATTERFIELD,
BREENA SATTERFIELD, ANNE M. SCHELL
AND CHRISTIANE M. HOPPE

EDITOR'S SYNOPSIS

The authors present data on an 8-year follow-up of 110 ADD hyperactive boys treated with drugs alone and 76 matched hyperactive boys treated with multimodal therapy (MMT). Records of arrest and institutionalization were found to be significantly lower in the MMT group. The annual cost of MMT is 1/10th that of institutionalization so that this is a cost-effective treatment approach for the prevention of delinquency in hyperactive boys. Obviously the damage to society and many individuals, including the patients themselves, of non-incarcerated antisocial personality disordered (ASPD) far exceeds that of the cost of incarceration.

In addition, the authors show the effects of social class and family settings on the development of ASPD from ADDH and normal children. (These effects were cancelled in the above study). In their study of family settings, e.g., natural family, one step-parent family, step-parent alone, the last group showed no manifestations of ASPD at the appropriate age of 18 years or over. ADD youths from broken families showed 2.7 times greater offender rates for one or more offenses than controls. For ADD youths from intact families, the offender rate for one or more offenses was 8 times higher for ADDH than controls; for multiple offenses it was more than 28 times higher, and for institutionalization it was more than 17 times higher (all exceeding $p < 0.001$).

A comparison of ADD youths with brothers of approximately the same age showed that the latter did not differ from normal controls. When the

ADD youths and their brothers were compared, it was found that the ADD offender rate for serious offenses was 4 times higher, for multiple serious offenses, it was 5 times higher, and for institutionalization, more than 34 times higher than for their brothers (at statistically significant rates).

Regrettably this chapter has been replaced by a summary because of publisher's demands and since a 10-year follow-up of the same group of children treated with drugs versus MMT appeared in: Satterfield JH, Satterfield BT, Schell AN: Therapeutic interventions to prevent delinquency in hyperactive boys. J. Amer. Acad. Child & Adolesc. Psychiat., 26:56–64, 1987.

Copies of the original chapter may be obtained from James H. Satterfield, M.D., National Center for Hyperactive Children, 5535 Balboa Boulevard, No. 215, Encino, CA 91316.

Index